Social Psychology and Health: European Perspectives

Edited by
D. R. RUTTER
LYN QUINE
Centre for Research in Health Behaviour
Department of Psychology
University of Kent at Canterbury

Avebury
Aldershot · Brookfield USA · Hong Kong · Singapore · Sydney

Published by
Avebury
Ashgate Publishing Ltd
Gower House
Croft Road
Aldershot
Hants. GU11 3HR
England

Ashgate Publishing Company
Old Post Road
Brookfield
Vermont 05036
USA

British Library Cataloguing in Publication Data
Social Psychology and Health: European
Perspectives
I. Rutter, D. R. II. Quine, Lyn
613
ISBN 1 85628 562 6

Library of Congress Cataloging-in-Publication Data
Social psychology and health : European perspectives / edited by D.R
Rutter and Lyn Quine
p. cm.
Based on a conference organized by the Centre for Research in Health Behaviour at the University of Kent at Canterbury, in Sept. 1991.
ISBN 1-85628-562-6 : £35.00 ($63.95 U.S. (approx.))
1. Health behaviour. 2. Health attitudes. 3. Health risk assessment. I. Rutter, D.R. (Derek R.) II. Quine, Lyn. III. University of Kent at Canterbury. Centre for Research in Health Behaviour. IV. European Association of Experimental Social Psychology.
RA776.9.S63 1994 94-27742
610'.1'9--dc20 CIP

Printed and Bound in Great Britain by
Athenaeum Press Ltd, Newcastle upon Tyne.

Contents

Figures and tables

List of contributors

Lars Åberg, Department of Psychology, Uppsala University, Box 1854, S-751 48 Uppsala, Sweden

Laurence Arnold, Centre for Research in Health Behaviour, Department of Psychology, University of Kent at Canterbury, Canterbury, Kent, CT2 7LZ, UK

Mark Conner, Department of Psychology, University of Leeds, Leeds, LS2 9JT, UK

Vera Hoorens, Department of Psychology, University of Groningen, Grote Kruisstraat 2/1, 9712 TS Groningen, The Netherlands

Gerjo Kok, Department of Health Education and Promotion, University of Limburg, PO Box 616, PL-6200 MD-Maastricht, The Netherlands

Neo Morojele, Department of Psychology, University of Kent at Canterbury, Canterbury, Kent, CT2 7LZ, UK

Paul Norman, Department of Psychology, University College of Swansea, Swansea, SA2 8PP, UK

Jos Poelman, STD Foundation, Utrecht, The Netherlands

Lyn Quine, Centre for Research in Health Behaviour, Department of Psychology, University of Kent at Canterbury, Canterbury, Kent, CT2 7LZ

Jo Reinders, National Centre of Health Education, Utrecht, The Netherlands

Derek Rutter, Centre for Research in Health Behaviour, Department of Psychology, University of Kent at Canterbury, Canterbury, Kent, CT2 7LZ

Herman Schaalma, Department of Health Education and Promotion, University of Limburg, PO Box 616, PL-6200 MD-Maastricht, The Netherlands

Paul Sparks, Biotechnology and Biological Sciences Research Council, Institute of Food Research, Reading Laboratory, Shinfield, Reading, RG2 9AT, UK

Geoffrey Stephenson, Department of Psychology, University of Kent at Canterbury, Canterbury, Kent, CT2 7LZ, UK

Stephen Sutton, Institute of Psychiatry, ICRF Health Behaviour Unit, 4 Windsor Walk, London, SE5 8AF, UK

Joop van der Pligt, Department of Social Psychology, University of Amsterdam, Roetersstraat 15, 1018 WB Amsterdam, The Netherlands

Preface

In September 1991, a small conference was organized by the Centre for Research in Health Behaviour at the University of Kent at Canterbury. It was held under the auspices of the European Association of Experimental Social Psychology, and it brought together leading social psychologists from Europe to discuss the role of social psychological theories and models in research on health behaviour. Three things soon became clear: the most widely used models came from the attitude and risk perception literatures; a great variety of behaviours were receiving empirical attention; and it would be useful to synthesize the diversity of approaches and findings in a book. Speakers were invited to write chapters around their talks, and one or two additional contributions were commissioned. This book is the result.

The opening chapters are concerned with attitudes. The first, by Conner and Norman, sets the scene by outlining the Health Belief Model and the Theory of Planned Behaviour, arguably the leading models in research on health attitudes and behaviour. They test the relative value of the models for predicting attendance at health screening. The second and third chapters, by Sparks and by Morojele and Stephenson, concentrate on the Theory of Planned Behaviour, and apply it to food choice and to addiction. Sutton, in Chapter 4, examines the role of previous behaviour in predicting present behaviour: does it have a direct effect or is there mediation, through beliefs and other cognitive dispositions; and is there a distinction to be drawn between habit and routine?

Chapters 5 and 6 mark a transition, for both use attitude models but are concerned with risk and safety. Chapter 5, by Åberg, applies the Theory of Planned Behaviour to drink-driving; and Chapter 6, by Arnold and Quine, re-examines the Health Belief Model and explores its implications for predicting and understanding helmet use among young cyclists. There then follow three chapters on perceptions of risk. In

Chapter 7, Van der Pligt reviews the recent literature on risk appraisal and health behaviour; in Chapter 8, Hoorens analyses the concept of unrealistic optimism and considers its implications for health behaviour; and in Chapter 9, Schaalma and his colleagues report on the development of AIDS education in Dutch secondary schools. In the final chapter, by Rutter and Quine, an attempt is made to draw the themes of the book together, and to argue for closer links between social psychology and epidemiology.

Any edited book is a collaborative effort. We are grateful to the European Association of Experimental Social Psychology for sponsoring the original meeting and to Avebury for agreeing to be the publishers; we are delighted with the quality of the chapters and the promptness with which they were delivered; and we continue to go ever deeper in debt to Jo Lemon, who edited the text, corrected the grammar and spelling, typed the camera ready copy, and so on, and so on, and so on.

Derek Rutter and Lyn Quine
May 1994

1 Comparing the Health Belief Model and the Theory of Planned Behaviour in health screening

Mark Conner and Paul Norman

Introduction

Health psychologists have long attempted to understand the factors that influence a health relevant decision. One set of factors that have received considerable attention are cognitive factors (e.g. Marteau, 1989). While a number of approaches might usefully be employed (Cummings et al., 1980), the Health Belief Model (HBM: Becker, 1974; Becker and Rosenstock, 1987) and the Theory of Planned Behaviour (TPB: Ajzen, 1985, 1988, 1991), which is a recent extension of the widely used Theory of Reasoned Action (TRA: Fishbein and Ajzen, 1975; Ajzen and Fishbein, 1980) have attracted interest from health psychologists. It is a comparison of these two cognitive models that forms the basis of this chapter.

Several studies have compared the HBM with the earlier TRA in the health area (Oliver and Berger, 1979; Mullen et al., 1987; Rutter, 1989). However, there have been no comparisons with the TPB in the health area (Conner and Norman, 1993). The principal advance of the TPB over the TRA is that it extends the TRA's area of application to non-volitional behaviours (Ajzen, 1988, 1991). This study compared the HBM and the TPB on the basis of their conceptual strengths and predictive validity in a study of health screening attendance behaviour. Ways in which variables from the two models might be combined in order to give better predictions of behaviour are also considered. Health screening was selected because it has been identified as an important way of detecting potential health risk factors and also of promoting healthier lifestyles. As such it represents an important health behaviour. Identifying the cognitive factors important to attendance may allow us to develop ways of improving attendance rates.

Health Belief Model

The Health Belief Model (HBM) (Figure 1.1) has been used in a wide range of health contexts, including preventive and screening activities, compliance with medical regimens, and responses to illness symptoms. Harrison et al. (1992) report finding over a hundred articles using the HBM. Generally these studies have been supportive of the applicability of the model, although the way it has been applied shows a great deal of variability between studies, leading some to conclude that it is more a collection of variables than a systematic theory (Conner, 1993; Schwarzer, 1992).

Briefly, the HBM postulates that an individual's decision about whether to follow a particular health related behaviour is determined by four psychological variables: perceived susceptibility, perceived severity, perceived benefits, and perceived barriers. First and second then, the likelihood of an individual deciding to take a health action is determined by his or her perception of his or her own susceptibility to, and the severity of, a particular condition or illness. So, the greater the perceived susceptibility and the perceived severity of the illness, the greater the likelihood of deciding to take action. Perceived susceptibility and severity are usually combined multiplicatively to give a measure of perceived threat.

The specific action taken is determined by a consideration of the perceived benefits of and barriers to various actions. Actions with many benefits and few barriers are most likely to be chosen. A final part of the model is a 'cue to action' (Janz and Becker, 1984). The cue may be internal, as in the case of perceived physical symptoms, or external, such as receiving an invitation to health screening. Becker (1974) has argued that certain individuals may be predisposed to respond to such cues because of the value they place on their health. Furthermore, Wallston and Wallston (1981) suggest that the extent to which individuals see their health to be under their own influence may also be a factor in health decisions. Hence, two other variables frequently added to the HBM are the value the individual places on health (Lau et al., 1986) and the individual's health locus of control beliefs, i.e. whether individuals consider their health to be under the control of internal factors, powerful others, or chance (Wallston and Wallston, 1981). Some researchers also suggest that intention to act is a mediating variable between the influencing variables in the HBM and behaviour (King, 1982; Calnan, 1984; Norman and Fitter, 1989). Hence a positive response to an invitation to attend screening should be apparent in both intention and behaviour measures. Studies that have addressed this issue offer some

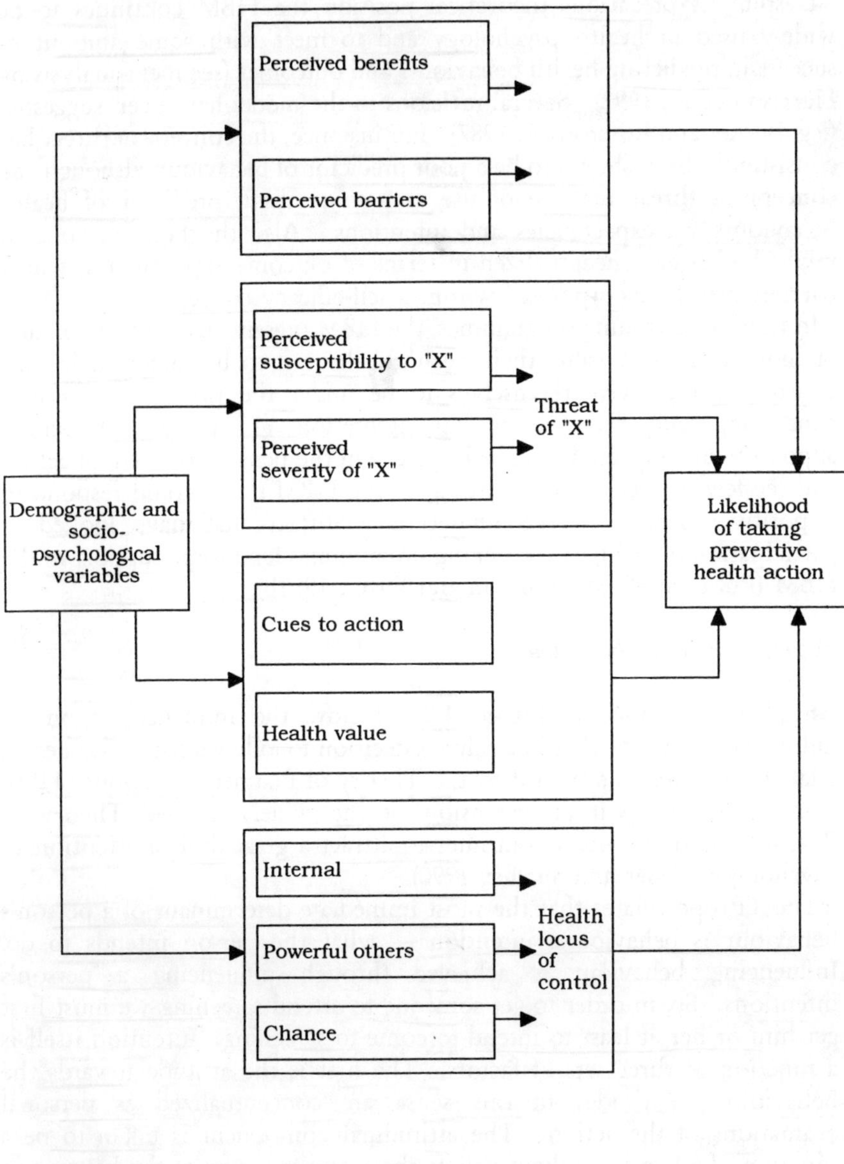

Figure 1.1 The Health Belief Model

limited support for this view (Calnan, 1984; King, 1982; Pill et al., 1988; Norman and Fitter, 1989).

Despite its precarious theoretical position the HBM continues to be widely used in health psychology and to meet with some amount of success in predicting health behaviours and outcomes (see meta-analysis by Harrison et al., 1992). Several revisions to the model have been suggested (e.g. Becker and Rosenstock, 1987). For instance, the concept of threat has consistently been shown to be a poor predictor of behaviour, although the concept of threat may be of use as a more distal predictor of health behaviours via expectancies and intentions. Also the benefits concept might be better conceptualized in terms of outcome expectancies, whilst barriers may be incorporated within a self-efficacy concept.

In terms of screening programmes, the HBM presents us with the picture of individuals who value their health, believe it to be under their own control, and perceive themselves to be under the threat of a serious condition, who then receive an invitation to attend a screening appointment. If these individuals believe in the benefits of such an action and see few barriers to it, according to the HBM they should respond in a positive manner to the invitation. Studies that have looked at participation in a range of screening programmes lend some support to the HBM (Pill et al., 1988; Norman and Fitter, 1991b).

Theory of Planned Behaviour

An alternative theory (Figure 1.2) of how the influences upon an individual determine that individual's decision to follow a particular health related behaviour is provided by the Theory of Planned Behaviour (TPB). This theory is itself an extension of the widely applied Theory of Reasoned Action, which continues to attract a great deal of attention in psychology (Tesser and Shaffer, 1990).

The TPB postulates that the most immediate determinant of a person's behaviour is behavioural intention – what the person intends to do. Influencing behaviour is achieved through influencing a person's intentions. So, in order to get someone to attend screening we must first get him or her at least to intend to come to screening. Intention itself is a function of three sets of factors. The first is the attitude towards the behaviour. Attitudes in this sense are conceptualized as personal evaluations of the action. The attitudinal component is taken to be a function of a person's salient beliefs about the outcome of the behaviour. These are conceptualized as being composed of an evaluation of each outcome of the behaviour multiplied by the strength with which each of health screening. Even the TRA has not been used extensively in the health field, although this has been advocated by some (Jaccard, 1975).

Differences and similarities between the HBM and TPB

Several differences and similarities become apparent when the two models are compared. The first difference is that the HBM predicts the actual probability of behaving in a particular way, while the TPB only predicts behaviour via behavioural intention. However, as noted above, several authors have found that placing intention between the predictors and behaviour improves the level of prediction of behaviour when using the HBM. This is in line with Becker et al. (1977) who have suggested that intention may intervene between variables in the HBM and health behaviour. This was also the approach taken here, allowing direct comparisons of the predictive power of the two models to be made.

A second difference is that the TPB examines individuals' beliefs and evaluations of the outcome of the behaviour. No evaluation of the outcome or consequences is required in the HBM: the outcomes of actions are assessed only as perceived benefits or barriers. A third difference is that the TPB considers individuals' perceptions of social norms/pressure, whereas normative influences in the HBM are simply listed among many other variables in the cues to action construct. Similarly, the TPB does not include aspects such as mass media messages, which are included in the cues to action component of the HBM. The TPB assumes that the variables listed under the cues to action (such as media messages, sociodemographic factors, etc.) are outside the model and only influence behaviour via their effects on behavioural beliefs and normative beliefs (Liska, 1984).

A final difference is that the HBM has separate components of perceived severity, susceptibility, and threat of the potential illness. The TPB, because it was developed in non-health related environments, does not explicitly cater for emotional fear and arousal variables. Consequently some have argued (Oliver and Berger, 1979) that the TRA (and so the TPB) is limited to the rational part of a health decision.

Several similarities between the two models are also apparent. Firstly, both models assess the likelihood of consequences. The HBM operationalizes this as benefits minus barriers, while the TPB uses outcome evaluations and facilitators and inhibitors to performance of the behaviour. Secondly, both models contain normative beliefs, as part of cues to action in the HBM and as part of subjective norm in the TPB. Thirdly, both models operationalize the extent to which the behaviour is under volitional control, the TPB as the perceived control component and the HBM as barriers to action.

A final similarity is in terms of the theoretical basis of both models – both are based on expectancy-value theory. Although the HBM does not explicitly state the rules for combining severity and susceptibility to predict perceived threat, many authors have used a multiplicative combination. In the TPB, expectancy-value theory dictates the multiplicative combination of outcome evaluation and belief strength, and normative beliefs and motivation to comply.

Objectives

To summarize, the major objective of this study was to compare the HBM and TPB in terms of their ability to predict intention and actual screening behaviour. A second objective was to examine the internal structure of the HBM and TPB to determine whether components of the two models could be combined to give better predictions of health screening behaviour.

Method

A total of 872 patients in a single rural practice in Norfolk, England were sent a copy of a questionnaire with items related to the HBM/TPB. After two mailings 47.9 per cent (N = 418) returned completed questionnaires. Of these patients, 407 were subsequently invited by a single letter for a health screening appointment during the following six months. Of the 407, 278 subsequently attended a health check and 129 failed to do so.

The measures

The Health Belief Model Perceived susceptibility and severity were measured by six items, each relating to six illnesses at which the health screening was particularly aimed. Rather than by separate measures, threat was assessed by multiplying the susceptibility and severity scores for each illness, as has been done in several other studies. Benefits and barriers were assessed by four and nine item scales derived from our previous research using the HBM to predict attendance at screening (Norman and Fitter, 1989, 1990, 1991a, 1991b). The cues to action variable, which has been measured in some studies of the HBM (Oliver and Berger, 1979), was not assessed because the invitation to screening sent to all patients was the specific cue to action. Health value was assessed by four items derived from previous studies (Norman, 1991; Norman and Fitter, 1991b). Three health locus of control dimensions (internal, powerful others, chance) were also measured, each by a four item scale based upon previous research (Norman, 1991; Wallston and Wallston, 1981). Each of these scales proved to have adequate reliability (Table 1.1).

The Theory of Planned Behaviour Salient beliefs and relevant referent groups were identified from our previous research on health screening (Norman and Fitter, 1989, 1990, 1991b) including semi-structured interviews with a number of patients (Norman and Fitter, 1991a). This procedure led to a total of four behavioural beliefs and eight referent groups. Attitudes were assessed on nine bipolar adjectives and subjective norms by a pair of items (Table 1.1). Behavioural control was assessed by two items. No direct independent measures of control beliefs were taken because of the overlap of these measures with the barriers concept in the HBM. Again all scales showed adequate internal reliability (Table 1.1).

Criterion variables Behavioural intention was assessed by a three item scale, while behaviour was based upon a dichotomous variable of attendance or non-attendance (Table 1.1).

Analyses

A series of reliable measures was first identified by a combination of exploratory and confirmatory factor analysis, and internal reliability measures were calculated (see Table 1.1). Simple correlation and regression analyses were then used to identify the best predictors of intention to attend an appointment and actual attendance at a health screening appointment. The regression analysis was essentially a form of path analysis (Duncan, 1975) with all antecedent variables regressed on to the criterion simultaneously in order to determine whether the independent variables would make a significant independent contribution to the explanation of variance in the criteria. This analysis method has been applied to comparisons of the HBM and TRA by other authors (Oliver and Berger, 1979).

Results

Behavioural intention was correlated with attendance behaviour. Although only a weak relationship was found ($r = 0.15$, $p < 0.01$), it is

Table 1.1
Reliability of scales from the HBM and TPB and representative items from each scale

	Items	Alpha	Representative items
Perceived Threat	6 x 2	0.86	Susceptibility x Severity to: weight problems, high blood pressure, cancer, heart disease, stroke, heart attack
Benefits	4	0.72	It's a good idea to have regular health checks Even if you think you are healthy, health checks are still a good idea
Barriers	9	0.92	I have children to take care of It would take up my spare time
Health Value	4	0.81	How important do you think it is that people take special care of their health? How often do you think about your health?
Internal HLOC	4	0.64	I am directly responsible for my health Whatever goes wrong with my health is my own fault
Powerful Others HLOC	4	0.70	Health professionals keep me healthy Following doctor's orders to the letter is the best way for me to stay healthy
Chance HLOC	4	0.60	Even if I take care of myself, it's easy to get ill When I become ill, it's a matter of fate
Attitudes	9	0.91	Attending a health check is: good-bad, harmful-beneficial, reassuring-worrying, unpleasant-pleasant
Behavioural Beliefs	4 x 2	0.84	A health check will help me learn to look after my health Learning how to look after my health is good
Subjective Norm	1 x 2	—	Advice to attend health check and desire to follow advice from people who are important to you
Normative Influence	8 x 2	0.91	Normative beliefs and motivation to comply with the following referent groups: spouse, other members of the family, closest friend, health experts, your doctor, the government, the media
Behavioural Control	2	0.55	I could easily attend a health check if I wanted to How much control have you over whether you attend a health check?
Intention	3	0.94	I intend to attend a health check if offered the opportunity If I were offered a health check I would try to attend

within the range of correlations reported in a recent meta-analysis of data on the TRA (Sheppard et al., 1988).

HBM results

The first part of Table 1.2 gives zero-order correlations between scores on the HBM scales and both the behavioural intention and behaviour measures. This shows that the simple correlations of these scales tended to be higher with intention than with behaviour, providing some support for the hypothesis that intention should be used in the HBM as an intervening variable between the predictor variables and behaviour.

The regression analysis (Table 1.3) for intention and behaviour revealed various significant beta coefficients. Intention was a function of benefits, barriers and health value. The perceived threat and the locus of control variables were not significant predictors of intention. This equation accounted for 55 per cent of the variability in the intention measure.

In the structural equation for behaviour no one variable was significant, and a non-significant proportion of variance in attendance behaviour was predicted (4 per cent). These data thus provide only partial support for the HBM. They do support the inclusion of a measure of health value in the model, though not health locus of control, but with intention as an intervening variable between the predictors and behaviour. Also, as is generally found in studies of health screening, perceived threat of illness is a poor predictor of attendance at screening.

TPB results

The second part of Table 1.2 gives the simple correlation of the scale scores with behavioural intention and behaviour. Again, the correlations with intention were higher than those with behaviour. The regression analysis for intention showed behavioural beliefs, attitudes and normative beliefs to be significant predictors, while subjective norm and behavioural control were non-significant predictors (Table 1.3). Together these variables predict 52 per cent of the variance in the intention measure, a similar proportion to that predicted by the HBM variables. The failure of behavioural control to predict intention indicates that this expansion of the TRA does not significantly improve the predictive power of the original model in the case of health screening attendance.

The results of the regression for behaviour are disappointing, explaining only a small, though significant, amount of variability in attendance behaviour (4 per cent). The only predictor to approach significance in this equation is normative beliefs (beta = – 0.17), which show a negative link

Table 1.2
Simple correlations between scales from the HBM and TPB and intention and attendance behaviour (N = 407)

	Intention	Behaviour
Intention	—	0.15**
HBM Scales		
Benefits	0.65**	0.15**
Barriers	0.55**	0.12**
Perceived threat	0.00	0.14
Internal HLOC	0.05	−0.01
Powerful others HLOC	0.17**	0.05
Chance HLOC	−0.13**	−0.03
Health value	0.45**	0.14**
TPB Scales		
Behavioural beliefs	0.51**	0.13*
Attitudes	0.68**	0.14**
Normative beliefs	0.52**	0.08
Subjective norm	0.57**	0.05
Behavioural control	0.41**	0.14**

* $p < 0.05$ ** $p < 0.01$

Table 1.3
Beta coefficients for the differing models

	Intention			*Behaviour*		
	HBM	TPB	Combined	HBM	TPB	Combined
R^2	0.55**	0.52**	0.61**	0.04	0.04*	0.05
Intention	—	—	—	0.03	0.10	0.04
HBM Scales						
Benefits	0.46**	—	0.33**	0.09	—	0.09
Barriers	0.29**	—	0.13**	0.04	—	0.03
Perceived threat	0.02	—	0.03	0.05	—	0.04
Internal HLOC	0.03	—	0.01	-0.02	—	-0.02
Powerful others HLOC	-0.01	—	-0.05	0.00	—	0.00
Chance HLOC	-0.03	—	0.00	-0.01	—	-0.03
Health value	0.20**	—	0.09*	0.08	—	0.09
TPB Scales						
Behavioural beliefs	—	0.19**	0.09*	—	0.07	0.03
Attitudes	—	0.45**	0.22**	—	0.05	0.00
Normative beliefs	—	0.15*	0.09	—	-0.17	-0.18
Subjective norm	—	0.05	0.06	—	0.07	0.08
Behavioural control	—	0.03	0.02	—	0.09	0.09

* $p < 0.05$ ** $p < 0.01$

with behaviour! This may be due to suppressor effects among variables. The other variables showed only weak links with behaviour.

Combining the HBM and TPB

Both models do explain statistically significant proportions of the variance in behavioural intention, suggesting that at least some of the antecedents of preventive health decisions have been identified. In addition, it may be possible to utilize non-redundant components from both models to improve prediction. The results of attempting such a combination of components for the HBM and TPB (Table 1.3) in predicting intention and behaviour indicate that taking variables from both models does improve the prediction of intention (61 per cent of variability), although not significantly. The statistically significant predictors of intention were benefits, barriers, health value, behavioural beliefs and attitudes.

The beta coefficients for behaviour were again disappointing with a non-significant proportion of variability being explained (5 per cent) and the only predictor to approach significance (normative beliefs, beta = – 0.18) likely to have been caused by suppressor effects.

Discussion

The study compared the HBM and TPB as predictors of intention to attend a health screening clinic and actual attendance. Simple correlations with intention were generally high and multiple regressions using variables from the HBM, TPB and both models combined accounted for 55 per cent, 52 per cent and 61 per cent of the variability in intention respectively. The significant predictors of intention were patients' behavioural beliefs and overall attitudes, perceived barriers and benefits of attendance, and health value. For actual behaviour, regressions were generally non-significant, but simple correlations suggested that the perceived benefits of screening and intentions to attend were the best predictors of attendance at health promotion screening clinics. Other important predictors were behavioural beliefs, attitudes, behavioural control, barriers, and health value. The practical implications of these findings are that in order to increase attendance at screening one would need to emphasize the benefits of screening or increase the intention to attend. On a theoretical note, it should be added that no evidence was found for perceived behavioural control being an independent predictor of intention, suggesting that the TPB may offer no improvement over the

TRA in predicting attendance at health screening (a behaviour under volitional control).

Comparing the two models revealed the HBM and TPB to be similar in predicting intention to attend screening and screening behaviour. Oliver and Berger (1979) found the TRA to be considerably superior to the HBM in predicting flu inoculation behaviour. Similarly Rutter (1989) reported the TRA to perform better than the HBM in predicting AIDS related behaviours. However, Mullen et al. (1987) like us reported that the TRA and HBM performed similarly in predicting changes in smoking, exercise and eating behaviours. The similar performance of the two models found here may be attributable to similarities between the variables that best predicted intention in the two models. The similarities between benefits and behavioural beliefs was noted earlier. Further similarities between health value concept and the outcome evaluation part of behavioural beliefs and between control beliefs and barriers is also worth noting.

Several studies have attempted to develop an integrative model of the cognitive influences upon behaviour (e.g. Mullen et al., 1987; Oliver and Berger, 1979). However, attempts to combine the variables from the two models were not particularly successful. The overlap between behavioural beliefs and benefits and also health value may mean that the two models are measuring overlapping constructs. The data do suggest the possible efficacy of including a barriers type of variable within the TRA/TPB. Similar suggestions have also been put forward by other authors (Norwich and Duncan, 1990) and it is interesting to note the similarity with the definition Ajzen (1991) gives for control beliefs. Conceptually a model that incorporates the best features of both models does appear possible. Schwarzer (1992) has proposed one such model in his health action process approach, but the superiority of such alternative conceptualizations has yet to be demonstrated empirically.

Despite these attempts to improve the predictive power of cognitive variables they continue to predict only a small proportion of the variability in attendance behaviour. Indeed, models of the influence of cognitive variables on health behaviours generally account for only a small proportion of variance in the behaviours studied. For instance, a meta-analytic study of the TRA in a range of diverse applications revealed about 10 per cent of studies to show correlations between behavioural intention and behaviour below 0.2 (Sheppard et al., 1988). The problem of the nature of the relationship between attitudes and behaviour has been a major focus of study in attitude research since Wicker's (1969) classic review. As Ajzen (1989) rightly points out, however, the relationship is not between two distinct variables, but between two indicators of a latent construct (the attitude): one verbal (attitude questionnaire), the other non-verbal (behaviour). There are a number of plausible reasons for the poor predictive power of cognitive models, which we will end by discussing.

Firstly, there may be a mismatch between the measures of the cognitive variables and behaviour. There are several aspects to this problem. In order for there to be a strong link between attitudes and behaviour the two must must be measured with the same level of specificity (Ajzen and Fishbein, 1974). Ajzen and Fishbein (1977) note the need to match the specificity of measurement of attitude and behaviour with respect to the target, the action, the time frame, and the situation. So, for instance, an individual's general attitude towards health care is likely to be a poorer predictor of his/her attendance at a specific health screening clinic than his/her specific attitude towards that particular health screening. While Ajzen and Fishbein (1977) emphasized the importance of matching the target and the action, a large gap in time between the measurement of attitudes and behaviour is also likely to weaken the attitude-behaviour link because of the possibility of attitude change during this time period, and differences in the situation may further weaken the relationship. Thus, failure to find a relationship between attitudes and behaviours towards the same attitude object may be due to a failure to match the specificity of the verbal and non-verbal measures of the attitude. However, it is worth noting that the specific attitude towards a particular behaviour is only one of many attitudes influencing the performance of that behaviour (and there are many other influences apart from attitudes). Indeed, attitudes towards one behaviour (e.g. work) are sometimes more significant in controlling other behaviours (e.g. attendance at screening) than the behaviour with which they are apparently concerned (Greenwald, 1989).

A final aspect of specificity which may have particularly affected this study is the lack of fidelity in the measurement of behaviour. The problems of using single items to measure psychological constructs are widely known and have led to the informed use of multi item scales (as used in this study). This psychometric principle has not been applied in general to the measurement of behaviour (Epstein, 1979, 1980). We should not even expect specific attitudes always to predict specific behaviours on specific occasions because, like single item scales, such behaviours are open to a whole range of idiosyncratic influences. Rather, specific attitudes should only be expected to measure specific behavioural tendencies when assessed over several occasions or situations in which the behaviour might be expected to occur. Recent books have devoted considerable space to this particular problem (Ajzen, 1988; Eagly and Chaiken, 1992). Moreover, studies by Fishbein and Ajzen (1974) and Weigel and Newman (1976) indicate that general attitudes predict general behaviours as measured by aggregate scores across several behavioural indices. Specific behaviours are held to be predicted by specific attitudes. What is being suggested here is that very specific behaviours when measured only on a single occasion may be so specific as to be particularly open to random influences, possibly distorting the relationship. Hence, the single offer of a screening appointment is likely to be influenced by a whole series of idiosyncratic events such as missing the bus on the way to the appointment or simply forgetting to attend. Thus the attendance measure may not truly reflect health screening behaviour if several opportunities to attend screening are offered. If such a measure of screening behaviour were available it would be predicted to correlate much more substantially with behavioural intention than it does in the current study. The problem of fidelity of measurement of the behaviour may similarly afflict other studies of the link between cognitive variables and health related behaviours, which frequently measure behaviour on a single occasion in a single context. This is not to contradict the need for specific attitude measures in order to predict specific behaviours, but merely to note that even specific attitude measures may not be at the same level of analysis as the individual behavioural act. The reliability of a specific act may be so low as to make it impossible to predict with any great reliability.

A second reason why cognitive models continue to account for such a small amount of variance in health related behaviours is that the models have been inadequately tested (Marteau, 1989). This may happen in at least three ways. Firstly, their constructs may be inadequately operationalized. This may be particularly relevant in relation to the HBM in which a multitude of operational definitions have been used across studies (Champion, 1984), often with scant regard to reliability and validity of the measures (Marteau, 1987). Oliver and Berger (1979) concluded that measurement is a problem with the HBM because it is more a collection of variables than a formal theory or model. It is not uncommon for studies of the same disease entity to operationalize the variables in the HBM differently.

Secondly, collected data may not always be analysed in accordance with the models' predictions. For example, in relation to the Health Locus of Control construct, Wallston and Wallston (1982) have argued that individuals' patterns of scores across the three dimensions should be considered rather than each dimension separately while, within the TPB, the way in which multiplicative composites such as belief strength x outcome evaluation are normally analysed using simple correlations has recently been criticized by Evans (1991).

Thirdly, the models may be misconceptualized by researchers. This is apparent with the TPB, which is primarily concerned with individuals' beliefs. Instead most researchers (including those in this study) supply modal belief statements and referent groups for respondents to rate, although there are notable exceptions (Rutter and Bunce, 1989; Rosin et al., 1992). The one comparison study of which we are aware (Rutter and Bunce, 1989) did find some support for the use of individually generated beliefs. Several studies have shown that individuals vary not only in the strength of their beliefs but in the salience of those beliefs to performance of a particular behaviour (Eiser and Van der Pligt, 1979; Budd, 1986; Van der Pligt et al., 1986). It may be that assessing non-salient beliefs produces distortions in the patterns of relationships among beliefs within the individual (see Wilson et al. 1989; Budd, 1987). Hence, collecting ratings of individually generated influences upon behaviour may be particularly important.

A third reason for the poor performance of the cognitive models most widely used in the health arena may centre on the models themselves. Firstly, it may be that they are not the best models from which to extract cognitive variables in order to predict health related behaviour. As Silver and Wortman (1980) point out, many of the models are not health specific and so may not be appropriate to use in the health area. In the present study this was true of the TPB, which does not cater for emotional arousal variables so important in health care decisions (Overall and Berger, 1979), possibly limiting its area of applicability to the rational side of a preventive health decision. However, the TPB did perform similarly to the more health specific HBM, possibly because of the overlap between the constructs that both models measure. Also, models may not adequately capture individuals' conceptualizations or representations of illness threats. The HBM, for example, employs a probabilistic approach to illness threat. However, Leventhal and Nerenz (1985) argue that individuals' reactions to illness are rather more concrete and categorical than is implied by the HBM, and that researchers should focus their attention on individuals' implicit models of illness. Also most of the models treat the influences upon health care decisions as static rather than part of an ongoing process (Schwarzer, 1992).

It may also be that the models provide an inappropriate conceptualization of the structure of individuals' attitudes and how these vary among individuals. As noted, the two models considered here use consensual beliefs, benefits, and so on, and they assume that differing influences are combined in a similar, linear, way within each individual. Research in other fields (e.g. consumer behaviour: Anderson, 1981) suggest that this may be an unrealistic assumption. An individualized methodology that allows individuals to generate their own behaviour-relevant influences, whatever they may be, and then analyses how they combine, may be particularly promising in increasing attitude-behaviour links. In addition, models that posit differing levels of information processing relevant to decisions (e.g. Petty and Cacioppo, 1986) may also be more widely applicable.

The fourth and final reason for the poor performance of the models is that other types of variables, not just cognitions, are important in the determination of health relevant behaviour. As they stand, most of the currently employed models are not placed in a wider context, and so do not consider broader social, economic and environmental influences on behaviour (Winett, 1985). Even the HBM, which includes demographic and sociopsychological variables, only includes them as modifying factors in the cues to action component. They are seen to have no more than an indirect influence on behaviour through their effect on individuals' cognitions. Furthermore, it can be argued that cognitive models of health related behaviour typically ignore the influence of past behaviour, or if its role is acknowledged it is usually through its effect on individuals' cognitions, which are still seen to be the primary determinants of behaviour. For instance, Ajzen (1988) suggests that any influence of previous behaviour in the TPB will act via the perceived control component. An exception to this trend has been the Bentler and Speckart (1981) attitude-behaviour model, which postulates a direct link between past behaviour and current behaviour. This type of model may prove to be more applicable in the health arena because, as Hunt et al. (1979) suggest, many health related behaviours are automatic and reflexive, with behaviours such as brushing one's teeth being a function of habit rather than cognitive variables (Allen and Taylor, 1984). To the extent that many health related behaviours can be seen to be habitual in nature, past behaviour may have a direct influence on current and future behaviour (Ronis et al., 1989). Abrams et al. (1991) have recently presented data indicating that such a model may indeed be more predictive than the TPB, at least for condom use. To the extent that many health related behaviours can be seen to be habitual in nature, past behaviour may have a direct influence on current and future behaviour.

Consideration of some of these issues may improve the predictive power of attitude models in health related behaviours. In particular, we believe that a focus on the measurement of health behaviours, further consideration of whether the most appropriate variables are being measured, and individualization of attitude measures in the health area are all warranted.

References

Abrams, D., Sheeran, P., Abraham, C. and Spears, R. (1991), 'Planned behaviour? Predicting condom-use with a new partner', paper presented at the BPS Social Section Conference, 20-22 September, 1991, University of Surrey.

Ajzen, I. (1985), 'From intentions to actions: a theory of planned behavior', in Kuhl, J. and Beckman, J. (eds), *Action Control: From Cognition to Behavior*, Springer, Heidelberg.

Ajzen, I. (1988), *Attitudes Personality and Behavior*, Open University Press, Milton Keynes.

Ajzen, I. (1989), 'Attitude structure and behavior', in Pratkanis, A.R., Breckler, S.J. and Greenwald, A.G. (eds), *Attitude Structure and Function*, Erlbaum, Hillsdale, NJ.

Ajzen, I. (1991), 'The Theory of Planned Behavior', *Organizational Behavior and Human Decision Processes*, 50, pp. 179-211.

Ajzen, I. and Fishbein, M. (1974), 'Factors influencing the intention-behavior relation', *Human Relations*, 27, pp. 1-15.

Ajzen, A. and Fishbein, M. (1977), 'Attitude-behavior relations: a theoretical analysis and review of empirical research', *Psychological Bulletin*, 84, pp. 888-918.

Ajzen, I. and Fishbein, M. (1980), *Understanding Attitudes and Predicting Social Behavior*, Prentice-Hall, Englewood-Cliff, NJ.

Allen, H.M. Jnr and Taylor, S.E. (1984), 'Alternative theories of health policy attitudes and protective behaviours: self interest, sociotrophy, and socialization', *Basic and Applied Social Psychology*, 5, pp. 19-35.

Anderson, N.H. (1981), *Foundations of Information Integration Theory*, Academic Press, New York.

Becker, M.H. (1974), 'The Health Belief Model and sick role behavior', *Health Education Monographs*, 2, pp. 409-419.

Becker, M.H., Haefner, D.P., Kasl, S.V., Kirscht, J.P., Maiman, L.A. and Rosenstock, I.M. (1977), 'Selected psychosocial models and correlates of individual health-related behaviors', *Medical Care*, 15 (supplement), pp. 27-46.

Becker, M.H. and Maiman, L.A. (1983), 'Models of health-related behavior', in Mechanic, D. (ed.), *Handbook of Health, Health Care and the Health Professions*, Free Press, New York.

Becker, M.H. and Rosenstock, I.M. (1987), 'Comparing social learning theory and the Health Belief Model', in Ward, W.B. (ed.), *Advances in Health Education and Promotion*, Vol. 2, JAI Press, Greenwich, CT.

Bentler, P. and Speckart, G. (1981), 'Models of attitude-behavior relations', *Psychological Review*, 86, pp. 452-264.

Budd, R.J. (1986), 'Predicting cigarette use: the need to incorporate measures of salience in the Theory of Reasoned Action', *Journal of Applied Social Psychology*, 16, pp. 663-685.
Budd, R.J. (1987), 'Response bias and the Theory of Reasoned Action', *Social Cognition*, 5, pp. 95-107.
Calnan, M. (1984), 'The Health Belief Model and participation in programmes for the early detection of breast cancer. A comparative analysis', *Social Science and Medicine*, 19, pp. 823-830.
Champion, V.L. (1984), 'Instrument development of the Health Belief Model constructs', *Advances in Nursing Science*, 6, pp. 73-85.
Conner, M.T. (1993), 'Pros and cons of social cognition models in health behaviour', *Health Psychology Update*, 14, pp. 24-31.
Conner, M.T. and Norman, P. (1993), 'Applying the Health Belief Model and Theory of Planned Behaviour to predicting attendance at health screening', in Dauwalder, J.P. (ed.), *Psychology and Promotion of Health*, Hogrefe and Huber, Lewiston, NY.
Cummings, M.K., Becker, M.H. and Maile, M.C. (1980), 'Bringing models together: an empirical approach to combining variables used to explain health actions', *Journal of Behavioral Medicine*, 3, pp. 123-145.
Duncan, O.D. (1975), *Introduction to Structural Equation Models*, Academic Press, New York.
Eagly, A.H. and Chaiken, S. (1992), *The Psychology of Attitudes*, Harcourt, Fort Worth, TX.
Eiser, J.R. and Van der Pligt, J. (1979), 'Beliefs and values in the nuclear debate', *Journal of Applied Social Psychology*, 9, pp. 524-536.
Epstein, S. (1979), 'The stability of behavior: I. On predicting most of the people most of the time', *Journal of Personality and Social Psychology*, 37, pp. 1097-1126.
Epstein, S. (1980), 'The stability of behavior: II. Implications for psychological research', *American Psychologist*, 35, pp. 790-806.
Evans, M.G. (1991), 'The problem of analyzing multiplicative composites: interactions revisited', *American Psychologist*, 46, pp. 6-15.
Fishbein, M. and Ajzen, I. (1974), 'Attitudes toward objects as predictors of single and multiple behavioral criteria', *Psychological Review*, 81, pp. 59-74.
Fishbein, M. and Ajzen, I. (1975), *Belief, Attitude, Intention, and Behavior*, Wiley, New York.
Greenwald, A.G. (1989), 'Why are attitudes important?', in Pratkanis, A.R., Breckler, S.J. and Greenwald, A.G. (eds), *Attitude Structure and Function*, Erlbaum, Hillsdale, NJ.

Harrison, J.A., Mullen, P.D. and Green, L.W. (1992), 'A meta-analysis of studies of the Health Belief Model with adults', *Health Education Research*, 7, pp. 107-116.

Hunt, W.A., Matarazzo, J.D., Weiss, S.M. and Gentry, W.D. (1979), 'Associative learning, habit, and health behavior', *Journal of Behavioral Medicine*, 2, pp. 111-124.

Jaccard, J. (1975), 'A theoretical analysis of selected factors important to health education strategies', *Health Education Monographs*, 3, pp. 152-167.

Janz, N.K. and Becker, M.H. (1984), 'The Health Belief Model: a decade later', *Health Education Quarterly*, 11, pp. 1-47.

King, J. (1982), 'The impact of patients' perceptions of high blood pressure on attendance at screening', *Social Science and Behaviour*, 16, pp. 1079-1091.

Lau, R.R., Hartman, K.A. and Ware, J.E. (1986), 'Health as a value: methodological and theoretical considerations', *Health Psychology*, 5, pp. 25-43.

Leventhal, H. and Nerenz, D. (1985), 'The assessment of illness cognition', in Karoly, P. (ed.), *Measurement Strategies in Health Psychology*, Wiley, New York.

Liska, A.E. (1984), 'A critical examination of the causal structure of the Fishbein/Ajzen attitude-behaviour model', *Social Psychology Quarterly*, 47, pp. 61-74.

Marteau, T.M. (1987), 'Health-related beliefs, attitudes and attributions: issues in measurement', *Proceedings of the Health Psychology Section, British Psychological Society*, pp. 32-37.

Marteau, T.M. (1989), 'Health beliefs and attributions', in Broome, A.K. (ed.), *Health Psychology: Processes and Applications*, Chapman and Hall, London.

Mullen, P.D., Hersey, J.C. and Iverson, D.C. (1987), 'Health behaviour models compared', *Social Science and Medicine*, 24, pp. 973-981.

Norman, P. (1991), 'Social learning theory and the prediction of attendance at screening', *Psychology and Health*, 5, pp. 231-239.

Norman, P. and Fitter, M. (1989), 'Intentions to attend a health screening appointment: some implications for general practice, *Counselling Psychology Quarterly*, 2, pp. 261-272.

Norman, P. and Fitter, M. (1990), 'Predicting attendance at health screening', paper presented at the Fourth European Health Psychology Society Conference, Oxford, 2-4 July 1990.

Norman, P. and Fitter, M. (1991a), 'Patients' views on health screening in general practice', *Family Practice*, 8, pp. 129-132.

Norman, P. and Fitter, M. (1991b), 'Predicting attendance at health screening: organisational factors and patients' health beliefs', *Counselling Psychology Quarterly*, 4, pp. 143-155.
Norwich, B. and Duncan, J. (1990), 'Attitudes, subjective norm, perceived preventive factors, intentions and learning science — testing a modified Theory of Reasoned Action', *British Journal of Educational Psychology*, 60, pp. 312-321.
Oliver, R.L. and Berger, P.K. (1979), 'A path analysis of preventive health care decision models', *Journal of Consumer Research*, 6, pp. 113-122.
Petty, R.E. and Cacioppo, J.T. (1986), 'The elaboration likelihood model of persuasion', in Berkowitz, L. (ed.), *Advances in Experimental Social Psychology*, Vol. 19, Academic Press, San Diego.
Pill, R., French, J., Harding, K. and Stott, N.C.H. (1988), 'Invitation to attend a health check in a general practice setting: comparison of attenders and non-attenders', *Journal of the Royal College of General Practitioners*, 38, pp. 53-56.
Ronis, D.L., Yates, J.F. and Kirscht, J.P. (1989), 'Attitudes, decisions, and habits as determinants of repeated behavior', in Pratkanis, A.R., Breckler, S.J. and Greenwald, A.G. (eds), *Attitude Structure and Function*, Erlbaum, Hillsdale, NJ.
Rosin, S., Tuorila, H. and Uutela, A. (1992), 'Garlic: a sensory pleasure or a social nuisance?', *Appetite*, 19, pp. 133-143.
Rutter, D.R. (1989), 'Models of belief-behaviour relationships in health', *Health Psychology Update*, 8-10 November, 1989.
Rutter, D.R. and Bunce, D.J. (1989), 'The Theory of Reasoned Action of Fishbein and Ajzen: a test of Towriss's amended procedure for measuring beliefs', *British Journal of Social Psychology*, 28, pp. 39-46.
Schwarzer, R. (1992), 'Self-efficacy in the adoption and maintenance of health behaviors: theoretical approaches and a new model', in Schwarzer, R. (ed.), *Self-efficacy: Thought Control of Action*, Hemisphere, London.
Sheppard, B.H., Hartwick, J. and Warshaw, P.R. (1988), 'The Theory of Reasoned Action: a meta-analysis of past research with recommendations for modifications and future research', *Journal of Consumer Research*, 15, pp. 325-339.
Silver, R.L. and Wortman, C.B. (1980), 'Coping with undesirable life events', in Garber, J. and Seligman, M.E.P. (eds), *Human Helplessness*, Academic Press, New York.
Six, B. and Schmidt, H. (1992), 'Overcoming a trauma: a meta-analysis of studies on the attitude-behavior relationship', paper presented at the 25th International Congress of Psychology, Brussels, 19-24 July, 1992.
Tesser, A. and Shaffer, D.R. (1990), 'Attitudes and attitude change', *Annual Review of Psychology*, 41, pp. 479-523.

Van der Pligt, J., Eiser, J.R. and Spears, R. (1986), 'Construction of a nuclear power station in one's locality: attitudes and salience', *Basic and Applied Social Psychology*, 7, pp. 1-15.

Wallston, K.A. and Wallston, B. (1981), 'Health locus of control scales', in Lefcourt, H. (ed.), *Research with the Locus of Control Construct*, Vol. 1, Academic Press, New York.

Wallston, K.A. and Wallston, B.S. (1982), 'Who is responsible for your health? The construct of health locus of control', in Sanders, G.S. and Suls, J. (eds), *Social Psychology of Health and Illness*, Erlbaum, Hillsdale, NJ.

Weigel, R.H. and Newman, L.S. (1976), 'Increasing attitude-behavior correspondence by broadening the scope of the behavioral measure', *Journal of Personality and Social Psychology*, 33, pp. 793-802.

Wicker, A.W. (1969), 'Attitudes versus actions: the relationship of verbal and overt behavioural responses to attitude objects', *Journal of Social Issues*, 4, pp. 41-78.

Wilson, T.D., Dunn, D.S., Kraft, D. and Lisle, D.J. (1989), 'Introspection, attitude change, and attitude-behavior consistency: the disruptive effects of explaining why we feel the way we do', in Berkowitz, L. (ed.), *Advances in Experimental Social Psychology*, Vol. 22, Academic Press, San Diego.

Winett, R.A. (1985), 'Ecobehavioral assessment in life-styles: concepts and methods', in Karoly, P. (ed.), *Measurement Strategies in Health Psychology*, Wiley, New York.

2 Food choice and health: Applying, assessing and extending the Theory of Planned Behaviour

Paul Sparks

Introduction

In this chapter, I offer an account of the application of Ajzen's Theory of Planned Behaviour (Ajzen, 1985, 1988, 1991) to the issue of food choice and discuss some empirical, methodological, and theoretical issues that the theory raises. The focus will be on research that my colleagues and I have carried out at the BBSRC Institute of Food Research, although reference will also be made to work in this area that has been reported by other authors. I shall adopt a rather more informal and discursive style than the standard journal format would permit in the hope of being able to raise a number of themes in a limited space (the reader is therefore recommended to refer to the cited texts for a more rigorous discussion of particular themes). Although the focus of the chapter will be on the Theory of Planned Behaviour in relation to food and health issues, a number of digressions are made to issues that bear on the more general application of the model and to perspectives that bear on similar themes (the model will not be outlined here, as it has already been described in the chapter by Mark Conner and Paul Norman).

Some introductory comments are in order. First, it is worth considering how food choice behaviour might or might not be distinctive when compared to other health related behaviours, such as those discussed in other chapters in this volume. Certainly in the western world, food choice is a ubiquitous and frequent activity. It is also an activity that is often characterized as involving a confrontation of competing motivations and ambivalent attitudes, 'weakness of the will', rapture and regret, indulgence and planned restraint. It is clearly not a social behaviour, in the sense that it necessitates social interaction, but it *is* often a social activity and social influences on choice are apparent both at interpersonal and broader structural levels (e.g. Bourdieu, 1984; Pill and Parry, 1989; Leather, 1992).

Second, although a link between diet and disease is widely acknowledged (Cannon, 1992), the health effects of *individual* food choice decisions are rarely as dramatically consequential as individual decisions about, for example, unprotected sex or drink-driving may be (cf. the chapters by Joop van der Pligt and Lars Åberg in this volume). The effects are generally more gradual and incremental.

Third, despite the general acceptance of the existence of a link between diet and health, disputes about dietary effects raise considerable ethical considerations for health promotion activities (Evans, 1988). Just as it is necessary to be aware of possible 'sins of commission' if health promotion activities are misdirected, so too is it necessary to recognize possible 'sins of omission' if no action is taken at all. And while the call for 'free and informed choice' is familiar within health promotion circles, it is all too easy to interpret this as a deceptive rhetoric for promotion strategies that verge on indoctrination. At the same time it needs to be recognized that vast sums of money are spent on advertising foods that can hardly be considered to be conducive to health: for example, it has been estimated that children in the US 'view an average of some 22,000 commercials per year, and more than 50 per cent of these advertise foods that are low in nutrition' (Logue, 1986, p. 99). In 1988, chocolate manufacturers spent £81.7 million on television advertising in the UK at the same time that the Government provided £4 million to the 'Look After Your Heart' campaign (Lang et al., 1989). Recognition of the individualistic bias apparent in health psychology (Becker, 1986) serves to alert attention to the broader social and economic influences on health behaviours: the usefulness of the kind of model discussed in this chapter therefore needs to be recognized as addressing but one level of explanation of behaviour in a complex network of causes and reasons.

The Theory of Reasoned Action, and its offshoot in the form of the Theory of Planned Behaviour, has been widely applied and its longevity has occurred despite some serious criticisms of the model which appeared soon after the publication of Ajzen and Fishbein's 1980 book. Criticism focused on the neglect of non-volitional behaviours and behaviours that involve social cooperation (Liska, 1984), and on the need to recognize the importance of the 'context of opportunity' in which actions are carried out (Sarver, 1983). Part of the reason for the basic model's longevity probably relates to its predictive power, despite the misgivings that many people express about its descriptive accuracy (cf. Fischhoff et al., 1982). I return to this problem below, but for now it is worth noting that many researchers are ambivalent about the use of the model because of these considerations. Another reason why the basic structure of the model has survived for so long is that it attacks the attitude-behaviour problem head on: it addresses one of the big issues in social psychology.

So, in advance of the conclusion to this chapter: what value the model? Well, it does predict: for example, highly significant correlations are generally found between summed belief-outcome evaluation products and attitudes, and between attitude and behavioural intentions. But then, on the other hand, as Becker (1986) suggests 'it's as easy to get correlations as it is to obtain calories' (p. 18). Clearly, the computational demands (i.e. summing the products of behavioural beliefs and outcome evaluations) that the model seems to propose as a descriptive account of attitude formation is a convenient fiction, introduced from the 'normative' proposals to be found in the decision making literature (e.g. Schoemaker, 1982). However, much of the attraction of the model rests with its direct reflection of the folk-psychological idea that people's attitudes will generally be reflected in their behaviour, providing behaviour is not coerced or otherwise constrained (this latter proviso is reflected to some extent in the 'perceived behavioural control' construct). While it is difficult to approach the model with anything but a generally critical attitude, this may be combined with enough intuitive faith in some of its basic premises to consider that development of the model is worthy of attention.

There is not the space in this chapter to go into a detailed account of the studies that will be referred to: rather the aim is to address some general issues that the use of this model raises. Specifically, this chapter briefly addresses five interrelated themes: within-subjects assessment, belief elicitation, attitude variability, applications of the model, and extensions to the model.

Within-subjects assessment

The origins of the Theory of Planned Behaviour in subjective expected utility theory from the decision making literature are clear and explicit (Ajzen and Fishbein, 1969; 1970). However, that tradition of analysing choice behaviour is based on the assessment of people's selection amongst alternative choice options. Such a 'within-subjects' application of the model has usually been eschewed in favour of an approach that correlates individuals' orderings on dimensions of attitudes and intentions (but see for example Davidson and Morrison, 1983). While we do not have a systematic programme of research addressing this within-subjects orientation, the data that we do have on this issue indicate stronger attitude-behaviour relationships when within-subjects choices are being investigated. For example, in a study of people's attitudes towards two flavoured milks (Shepherd, Sparks, Bellier and Raats, 1993), it was found that while the correlation between attitudes and intentions was 0.58 and 0.53 for the two milks independently, the correlation between differential attitude[1] and differential intention was 0.73. Raats (1992) reports a similar pattern of findings in a study of attitudes towards milks of different fat contents.

Assessing beliefs, outcome evaluations, and attitudes for a number of behavioural alternatives obviously requires a tremendous investment of research input to a questionnaire or survey procedure (and may impose unreasonable demands on 'subjects'). But multiple behavioural alternatives are often available in choice situations and it seems reasonable that research methods should reflect this in some way. In the context of food choice, as with other behaviours, these alternatives are often not mutually exclusive; abstinence is often also an option, at least in the short term.

However, the descriptive inaccuracy of the computationally complex summation of belief and outcome evaluation products has already been noted: more attention needs to be paid to the actual decision making strategies that people use in different choice situations and how these strategies influence attitudes. Payne, Bettman and Johnson's (1992) observation from accumulating evidence that 'when faced with multi-alternative decision tasks, people prefer noncompensatory choice strategies' (p. 98) would seem to support this suggestion. From another perspective, Dan-Cohen (1992) suggests a contrast between *willing* and *choosing*:

> I can sometimes approach the restaurant menu with a very specific craving for lobster: I'm not really interested in what's on the menu, other than to verify that lobster is still on it. It's not quite the case that at this point I prefer lobster to all other foods: I do not consider any other food at all. (p. 229)

For our interests in understanding food choice, we are keen to find out more about the processes of attitude formation in different situations and the extent to which these correspond to, and how they differ from, the very analytic, systematic and 'compensatory' process described within the Theory of Reasoned Action/Planned Behaviour.

Belief elicitation

While extensive within-subjects questionnaire designs are time consuming, they remain more faithful to the structure of choice situations than does simple between-subjects correlational assessment of single behaviours. A similar methodological problem arises with elicitation of the behavioural beliefs that are incorporated into the questionnaires used to assess the model. There is a clear distinction made in Ajzen and Fishbein's (1980) book between the measurement of individual salient beliefs and modal salient beliefs in the application of the model (pp. 62-73). Presumably because of the increase in research investment that it involves, the use of individuals' beliefs has been less commonplace than the use of modal salient beliefs. Rutter and Bunce's work on attitudes towards milk consumption (1989) is a rare exception to this (but see Rosin, Tuorila and Uutela, 1992; Sparks and Shepherd, in preparation (a)) even though the method appears to be on a firmer theoretical footing than the method of assessing modal salient beliefs. At an empirical level, the method seems especially advantageous where a diverse range of beliefs about the attitude 'object' are apparent. That method also avoids some awkward scaling issues that are involved when modal salient beliefs are used (Hewstone and Young, 1988; Sparks, Hedderley and Shepherd, 1991).

The standard belief elicitation procedure is provided in Ajzen and Fishbein (1980, pp. 63-4). Essentially, it involves asking subjects about the advantages and disadvantages of carrying out the behaviour in question. However, there are potential pitfalls with the method. First, it may elicit a sample of responses that is biased towards 'cognitive' influences, in much the same way that Wilson et al. (1989) suggest is the case when people are asked to explain their feelings:

> When people think about why they feel the way they do, we suggest that they feel compelled to give a 'good story' to explain their feelings. The reasons they come up with emphasize cognitions about the attitude object, and the reasons are often incomplete or incorrect. Further, these cognitions often consist of a biased sample of reasons that imply a different attitude than the one subjects previously held. Unaware that their reasons are a biased sample, subjects change their attitude in the direction implied by their reasons. Because the reasons consist of beliefs about the attributes of the attitude object, this new attitude has a heavy cognitive flavor. Behavior often remains affectively driven, however, resulting in reduced attitude-behavior consistency. (pp. 288-289)

Although the importance of affective (e.g. Ajzen and Driver, 1991) and experiential (Zanna and Rempel, 1988) aspects of attitudes has received recent attention, the implications for belief elicitation procedures have as yet not been addressed in the literature.

A second problem with standard elicitation procedures is that they may elicit the more easily articulated influences on attitudes, while influences that are more difficult to articulate, (e.g. affective, moral, self-identity [see below]), which may in fact be important influences on attitudes and behaviour, may be under-represented. This is certainly the impression that we have from our own research. It may be the case that alternative methods for eliciting behavioural beliefs, such as developments based on the repertory grid technique (Raats, 1992), provide an improvement on current techniques, but this remains to be demonstrated. This issue is important for health promotion concerns which seek to follow one implication of the Theory of Planned Behaviour: namely, that in order to change behaviour, it is advisable to address influences on attitudes (such as, and especially, behavioural beliefs). Certainly there is evidence in the food choice literature that 'sensory' ratings of foods may have an influence on consumption intentions that is independent of the contribution of attitudes towards consumption (Tuorila-Ollikainen, Lähteenmaki and Salovaara, 1986; Shepherd, Sparks, Bellier and Raats, 1993). For example, Torulae-Ollikainen et al. found that sensory evaluations of low-salt bread contributed to the prediction of consumption intentions independently of the contribution of attitudes.

Attitude variability

A major 'problem' for SEU models/rational models of choice has been the fact that people have variable or 'inconsistent' preferences (e.g. March, 1978), or they may express different attitudes at different times. The careful 'weighing up' of outcomes has already been noted as largely fictional; rather, different outcomes and issues may become salient at different times. Alternatively, even if people do weigh up different outcomes,or different pros and cons, they may not arrive at a composite attitudinal judgement: they may remain essentially ambivalent. In the context of food choice, such ambivalences are often very apparent: this has been noted by researchers from different perspectives (in addition to being a familiar experience to many). Ainslie (1986) discusses some of the 'precommitting devices' that people may use to cope with the influence of short term interests. Eagly and Chaiken (1993) note a number of potential influences on attitudes (see for example p. 209) which pave the way for various possible conflicts. White and Wetherell (1988), from a perspective that has emphasized the importance of variability in discourse, point to the conflict between desires to be slim and to avoid being a 'fashion victim', and how dieting may be accounted for by ('legitimate') health related motives.

One of the major problems that is often noted with the Theory of Reasoned Action/Planned Behaviour is that for the model to work accurately the time interval between the components needs to be small. In reality, various contextual factors can impinge upon the components of the model to alter attitudes and intentions. In one of our studies (Sparks, Hedderley and Shepherd, 1992), people were asked to report the extent to which their feelings about consuming wholemeal bread and biscuits varied and whether their feelings about consuming these items differed at different times. First, subjects reported more variability in their attitudes towards biscuits than they did towards wholemeal bread. Second, there was some evidence that higher variability was associated with reduced relationships between model components (see Table 2.1).[2]

This is of interest to us for theoretical reasons since it hints at a considerable flux in the psychological constructs that represent the main components of the model. Also of interest, however, from a concern with the relationship between diet and health, is to examine the factors that influence this variability: for example, to examine how sensory appeal and health concerns become salient themes under different contextual conditions. How is it that future consequences (e.g. good health) may often be disregarded in favour of more immediate (e.g. sensory) benefits? Herrnstein (1990), for example, notes how we discount deferred consequences of acts when we make choices and he talks about our 'ubiquitous tendency to be overinfluenced by imminent events' (p. 358). 'Imagine', he suggests,

> that we could always select meals for tomorrow, rather than for right now. Would we not all eat better than we do? We may find it possible to forego tomorrow's chocolate cake or second helping of pasta or third martini, but not the one at hand. (p. 359)

This would indicate that the temporal proximity of behavioural outcomes influences the value placed on those outcomes at different time points. But 'temporal proximity' in itself is not a sufficient psychological explanation: more attention needs to be paid, for example, to the processes by which desires, preferences, and attitudes undergo change (cf. Hoch and Loewenstein, 1991). These issues are very pertinent for the understanding of food choice.

Table 2.1
Comparison of higher and lower variability groups (probability values are based on one-tailed tests of significance)

	Variability					
	Higher		Lower			
	r	n	r	n	Z_{obs}	
Wholemeal bread consumption						
Attitude-intention[1]	0.54	85	0.72	81	−1.94	*
Attitude-intention[2]	0.47	85	0.47	81	0.04	
Attitude-desire[1]	0.76	85	0.74	81	0.35	
Attitude-desire[2]	0.75	85	0.78	81	−0.46	
Attitude-expectation[1]	0.54	85	0.76	81	−2.47	**
Attitude-expectation[2]	0.49	84	0.48	81	0.16	
Past behaviour-intention[2]	0.83	83	0.93	79	−2.93	**
Past behaviour-desire[2]	0.47	83	0.61	79	−1.20	
Past behaviour-expectation[2]	0.85	82	0.94	79	−3.00	**
Biscuit consumption						
Attitude-intention[1]	0.32	79	0.41	86	−0.66	
Attitude-intention[2]	0.32	80	0.57	84	−1.94	*
Attitude-desire[1]	0.28	80	0.53	85	−1.90	*
Attitude-desire[2]	0.42	80	0.59	86	−1.49	
Attitude-expectation[1]	0.17	80	0.49	86	−2.35	**
Attitude-expectation[2]	0.24	80	0.59	85	−2.68	**
Past behaviour-intention[2]	0.52	79	0.90	82	−5.38	***
Past behaviour-desire[2]	0.42	79	0.61	84	−1.61	
Past behaviour-expectation[2]	0.48	79	0.91	83	−6.13	***

Intention[1] = intention to eat during next week
Intention[2] = amount intended to eat tomorrow
Expectation[1] = expectation of eating during next week
Expectation[2] = amount expected to eat tomorrow
Desire[1] = wish to eat during next week
Desire[2] = wish to eat tomorrow

* $p < 0.05$ ** $p < 0.01$ *** $p < 0.0001$

Applications of the Theory of Planned Behaviour

There have been a number of successful applications of the Theory of Planned Behaviour (see Ajzen, 1991, Table 1) including, in the context of food choice, studies by Beale and Manstead (1991); Sparks, Hedderley and Shepherd (1992); and Sparks, Shepherd, Wieringa and Zimmermanns (submitted). This indicates that the perception of control problems of one sort or another seems to be adding to the predictive capacity of the Theory of Reasoned Action structure. But this kind of assessment tells us that control problems are likely to be influential for intentions and behaviour but does not tell us what these control problems are. In order to examine this latter issue in the context of food choice, we are interested in assessing the factors that influence perceived behavioural control. *If* we need to know about people's beliefs and values in order to influence attitude change, then we also need to know about the nature of the control problems that people experience in order to address those kinds of influences upon behaviour too. We have sought in pilot work to elicit some indication of the control problems that influence consumption of particular foods. The aim has then been to incorporate measures assessing these control problems into questionnaires and to use them to enable a prediction of perceived behavioural control. Table 2.2 shows some of the relationships that we have discovered.

Although in all of these cases we are not managing to explain much of the variance in perceived behavioural control, some method of this sort seems to be worth pursuing. Recently Ajzen has begun to examine the underpinnings of perceived behavioural control through an examination of *control beliefs* and *power* (Ajzen, 1991; Ajzen and Driver, 1991). We have followed this lead in assessing similar issues (Sparks and Shepherd, in preparation (b)). However, in pursuing this goal, we often experience difficulties (!) with inter-item reliability when measuring perceived control (see Table 2.3), and a similar problem has been reported by other authors (e.g. Beale and Manstead, 1991). We are unclear at the moment about the reasons for this, although the difference between unipolar and bipolar response scales may well be a confounding factor, as may a distinction in the public mind between *control* and *difficulty* (in which terms perceived behavioural control items are typically couched). Of course, questionnaire context effects (e.g. Budd, 1987) may also be contributory factors.

Table 2.2
Regressions of perceived behavioural control on predictor variables (reflecting potential problems of control) elicited from pilot work

	R	R^2	Predictor variable	Beta
PBC: Wholemeal bread consumption (Sparks, Hedderley and Shepherd, 1992)	0.49	0.24	Availability	−0.09
			Cost	−0.25 **
			Resisting	−0.02
			Others' preference	−0.31 ***
PBC: Biscuit consumption (Sparks, Hedderley and Shepherd, 1992)	0.46	0.21	Availability	−0.05
			Cost	−0.14
			Resisting	−0.44 ***
			Others' preference	−0.08
PBC: Organic vegetable consumption (Sparks and Shepherd, 1992)	0.23	0.05	Availability	−0.17 *
			Cost	−0.03
			Family influence	−0.11
			Friends' influence	−0.13

* $p < 0.05$ ** $p < 0.01$ *** $p < 0.001$

Table 2.3
Perceived behavioural control measures: inter-item reliability

Reference	Attitude issue	Number of PBC items	Cronbach's alpha
Sparks, Hedderley and Shepherd (1992)	Consumption of wholemeal bread	2	0.43
Sparks, Hedderley and Shepherd (1992)	Consumption of biscuits	2	0.55
Sparks and Shepherd (1992)	Consumption of organic vegetables	3	0.65

Extensions to the Theory of Planned Behaviour

Having successfully introduced a measure of perceived behavioural control into the model structure, Ajzen has recently indicated that the addition of other factors may improve the predictive capabilities of the model:

> The theory of planned behavior is, in principle, open to the inclusion of additional predictors if it can be shown that they capture a significant proportion of the variance in intention or behavior after the theory's current variables have been taken into account. (1991, p. 199).

One such modification to which Ajzen alludes is the inclusion of a measure of perceived moral obligation (or 'moral norm'), and he cites a study of lying, cheating and stealing behaviour (Beck and Ajzen, 1991), which showed the importance of the inclusion of such a measure. This variable has received sporadic attention in the literature (e.g. Schwarz, 1978; Gorsuch and Ortberg, 1983; Zuckermann and Reis, 1978) and is one that Ajzen and Fishbein note but to which they pay only scant attention in their 1980 book (see p. 247). We have recently had some success in incorporating this variable into research investigating attitudes towards the use of gene technologies in food production: technologies that clearly raise a number of ethical issues. For example, in a study of attitudes towards the application of gene technology (also known as genetic engineering), the role of a measure of perceived ethical obligation to support or oppose the use of the technology was examined (Sparks, Shepherd and Frewer, in press). Regressions of expectations of supporting the technology on attitudes, subjective norm, perceived behavioural control and perceived moral obligation revealed a marginally significant independent effect for a measure of perceived moral obligation. A similar effect was found for a regression of expectations of eating food produced using the technology. Moreover, this study showed predictive effects of a measure of obligation on *attitudes*, independent of the contribution of $\Sigma b \times e$ (see Table 2.4). Likewise, Raats (1992) has shown that people's feelings of obligation for their family's health may influence intentions to use milk, independently of their attitudes towards use (Raats, 1992): here again, measures of obligation also revealed an independent effect on attitudes. These findings may be seen as congruent with Eagly and Chaiken's (1993) suggestion that attitudes will be influenced by factors other than utilitarian ones (cf. Sparks, 1993).[3]

Many social behaviours involve moral issues, and the role of reasoning about moral issues within a framework such as that of the Theory of Planned Behaviour needs further attention, especially in relation to the

Table 2.4
Regressions of (a) expectations of eating food produced by gene technology and expectations of supporting the use of technology in food production, and (b) attitudes towards eating food produced by gene technology and attitudes towards supporting the use of the technology in food production

Predictor variable	R	R^2	Increment	F_{change}	Final Beta
Expectation of eating food produced by the technology					
Attitude	0.39	0.15	0.15	28.6	0.23 *
Others' attitudes					0.14
Perceived control	0.41	0.17	0.02	6.9	- 0.14 **
Self-identity	0.43	0.18	0.01	4.6	0.12 *
Perceived ethical obligation	0.44	0.19	0.01	3.6	- 0.12 †
Expectation of supporting use of the technology in food production					
Attitude	0.88	0.77	0.77	542.1	0.77 ***
Others' attitudes					0.06
Perceived control	0.88	0.77	0.00	0.0	0.00
Self-identity	0.88	0.77	0.00	0.8	-0.02
Perceived ethical obligation	0.88	0.78	0.00	3.5	0.08 †
Attitude towards eating food produced by the technology					
$\sum b \times e$	0.67	0.44	0.44	224.1	0.46 ***
Perceived ethical obligation	0.76	0.57	0.13	84.9	- 0.41 ***
Attitude towards supporting use of the technology in food production					
$\sum b \times e$	0.66	0.44	0.44	223.3	0.33 ***
Perceived ethical obligation	0.83	0.69	0.25	221.4	0.60 ***

† $p < 0.10$ * $p < 0.05$ ** $p < 0.01$ *** $p < 0.001$

SEU basis of the model and the usefulness of 'utility' based theories of choice (see Sparks, 1993). Certainly there seems to be no *prima facie* reason why people's expressed attitudes should not be influenced by moral considerations. Not surprisingly, the moral dimension to food choice has been addressed from perspectives other than the one described here (e.g. Beardsworth and Keil, 1992).

Another suggested modification to the Theory of Reasoned Action that has received some recent attention is that a measure of self-identity could make a contribution to the prediction of intentions that is independent of the contribution provided by attitudes (Biddle, Bank and Slavings, 1987; Charng, Piliavin and Callero, 1988). We were interested in these findings, although we did not find the presented arguments for the hypothesized effects to be very convincing. In particular, we did not feel that there was a strong case for expecting independent effects of attitudes and self-identity. Consequently, we conducted some research of our own: a study of attitudes towards the consumption of organically produced vegetables in which we included a measure of self-identification as a 'green consumer' (Sparks and Shepherd, 1992). What we found, much to our surprise, was a significant contribution of the self-identity measure when we regressed intentions on the other relevant model components (see Table 2.5).

Since we thought that self-identity might simply act as some kind of proxy for past behaviour, we included a measure of past consumption as an additional predictor variable in the regression: however, the significant effect for the self-identity measure persisted. We have recently extended this line of investigation in a study of attitudes towards fat reduction in which a measure of identification 'as someone concerned about the health consequences of what I eat' again resulted in independent effects on behavioural expectations (Sparks, Shepherd, Wieringa and Zimmermanns, submitted). However, a similar measure on a similar topic in a separate study did not reveal an independent 'self-identity' effect (Sparks, Shepherd, Wieringa and Zimmermanns, 1992).

As well as this potential addition to the structure of the Theory of Planned Behaviour being of considerable theoretical importance (see Eagly and Chaiken, 1993), from a concern with food choice and health there are also immediate practical issues at stake. For example, the image of 'healthy eating' and the identities that accompany it may influence the uptake, or otherwise, of dietary habits that are conducive to good health. 'Healthy eating' may no longer be the prerogative of 'cranks' and 'faddists' (cf. Murcott, 1988) but the symbolism of healthy eating may be expected to influence behaviour. Bourdieu (1984), for example, discusses not only how the different consequences of food consumption may be differently valued by different social classes, but also how 'taste classifies, and it

Table 2.5

Regressions of intentions to consume organic vegetables on attitudes, subjective norm, perceived control and self-identity

Predictor variable	R	R^2	Increment	F_{change}	Final Beta
Attitude					0.21 **
	0.41	0.17	0.17	21.6	
Subjective norm					0.16 *
Peceived control	0.49	0.24	0.06	17.4	0.26 ***
Self-identity	0.52	0.27	0.04	11.0	0.22 **

* $p < 0.05$ ** $p < 0.01$ *** $p < 0.001$ df = 210

classifies the classifier' (p. 6), implying the involvement of a myriad of social categorization issues.

In 1980, Ajzen and Fishbein suggested of the Theory of Reasoned Action: 'The accumulating evidence suggests ... that the theory is useful for most individuals and with respect to most social behaviors' (p. 245). Useful, perhaps, in the sense of predicting attitudes, intentions and behaviour from their respective 'proximal determinants' for many behaviours. But it apparently was not sufficient for many social behaviours of interest, since the introduction of a measure of perceived behavioural control into the structure of the model has met with impressive predictive success (e.g. Ajzen, 1991). While many social behaviours of interest clearly involve, to some extent, problems of control, many social issues are also moral issues, and the increased attention recently paid to moral dimensions represents a clear indication of a further useful extension to the basic model.

Concluding comments

In this chapter I have been able to provide only a very brief indication of applications of the Theory of Planned Behaviour in the domain of food choice. Some misgivings about the theory have been aired and some indication has been given of areas where further research using the model could be profitably targeted. It has been possible to ignore a number of important themes (such as the role of habit, of anticipatory regret, and the application of more sophisticated statistical methods) only because these have been developed by other contributors to this volume.

The Theory of Planned Behaviour has a number of limitations but it does offer the basis for addressing some important food and health issues. As well as applying the model, 'tinkering' with it, adding components and increasing percentage variance accounted for, it is also worthwhile to examine problems for the model: to look at cases where it does not apply, or where it performs badly, and how the lessons learned there can be used productively. These are all useful pursuits. However, with a view to health promotion concerns, we need to assess the model as a basis for researching attitude change, persuasion and information provision. As we are interested in assisting with the promotion of dietary change, we want to know about the origins of people's beliefs, values, and attitudes and about the control problems that people experience in making such changes; and we want to understand more about the processes of change.

Finally, it is apparent that the application of the model to practical issues such as health promotion concerns presents the opportunity for a symbiosis between 'pure' and 'applied' research. Learning of the experience of researchers in other health related domains invariably offers fresh insights. Reflection on other models and approaches (such as those presented elsewhere in this volume) presents a confrontational challenge where competing perspectives are offered, and the opportunity for integration where perspectives are essentially complementary. Largely under the impetus from contributions to this volume, for example, my colleagues and I have recently begun to address the role of 'unrealistic optimism' and affective factors, such as regret, in the context of food choice issues, and how these might be incorporated into applications of the Theory of Planned Behaviour (Sparks, Shepherd, Wieringa and Zimmermanns, submitted; Sparks and Shepherd, in preparation (b)). At another level, it is also helpful to examine the perspectives of other disciplines and different forms of explanation in order to further our understanding of food choice issues.

Eagly (1992) has recently commented that 'The popularity of these expectancy-value models in applied research is unprecedented in social psychology' (p. 695). To date, the Theory of Planned Behaviour has featured heavily in our research work and we consider it to be a useful basis on which to explore food choice and health issues. While Wolfgang Stroebe once suggested that theories in social psychology typically undergo change 'due to satiation rather than refutation', there is certainly little sign at the moment of researchers losing their appetite for the central premises of this particular model.

Notes

1. Taken as the difference between the two attitude measures.

2. It should be noted here that Norman and Smith (submitted) have recently failed to replicate this finding in a study of exercise behaviour. Though some of the differences examined matched the predicted direction, these differences were not statistically significant.

3. Although Eagly and Chaiken are unclear about how 'utilitarian' behavioural outcomes are to be distinguished from other behavioural outcomes.

References

Ainslie, G. (1986), 'Beyond microeconomics. Conflict among interests in a multiple self as a determinant of value', in Elster, J. (ed.), *The Multiple Self*, Cambridge University Press, Cambridge.

Ajzen, I. (1985), 'From intentions to actions: a theory of planned behavior', in Kuhl, J. and Beckmann, J. (eds), *Action Control: From Cognition to Behavior*, Springer, Berlin.

Ajzen, I. (1988), *Attitudes, Personality and Behaviour*, Open University Press, Milton Keynes.

Ajzen, I. (1991), 'The Theory of Planned Behaviour', *Organizational Behaviour and Human Decision Processes*, 50, pp. 179-211.

Ajzen, I. and Driver, B.L. (1991), 'Prediction of leisure participation from behavioral, normative, and control beliefs: an application of the Theory of Planned Behavior', *Leisure Sciences*, 13, 3, pp. 185-204.

Ajzen , I. and Fishbein, M. (1969), 'The prediction of behavioral intentions in a choice situation', *Journal of Experimental Social Psychology*, 5, pp. 400-416.

Ajzen, I. and Fishbein, M. (1970), 'The prediction of behavior from attitudinal and normative variables', *Journal of Experimental Social Psychology*, 6, pp. 466-487.

Ajzen, I. and Fishbein, M. (1980), *Understanding Attitudes and Predicting Social Behaviour*, Prentice-Hall, Englewood Cliffs, New Jersey.

Ajzen, I. and Madden, T.J. (1986), 'Prediction of goal-directed behavior: attitudes, intentions and perceived behavioral control', *Journal of Experimental Social Psychology*, 23, pp. 453-474.

Beale, D.A. and Manstead, A.S.R. (1991), 'Predicting mothers' intentions to limit frequency of infants' sugar intake: testing the Theory of Planned Behavior', *Journal of Applied Social Psychology*, 21, 5, pp. 409-431.

Beardsworth, A. and Keil, T. (1992), 'The vegetarian option: varieties, conversions, motives and careers', *The Sociological Review*, pp. 253-293.

Beck, L. and Ajzen, I. (1991), 'Predicting dishonest actions using the Theory of Planned Behaviour', *Journal of Research in Personality*, 25, pp. 285-301.

Becker, M.H. (1986), 'The tyranny of health promotion', *Public Health Reviews*, 14, pp. 15-23.

Biddle, B.J., Bank, B.J. and Slavings, R.L. (1987), 'Norms, preferences, identities and retention decisions', *Social Psychology Quarterly*, 50, 4, pp. 322-337.

Bourdieu, P. (1984), *Distinction: A Social Critique of the Judgement of Taste*, Routledge and Kegan Paul, London.

Budd, R.J. (1987), 'Response bias and the Theory of Reasoned Action', *Social Cognition*, 5, 2, pp. 95-107.

Cannon, G. (1992), *Food and Health: The Experts Agree*, London, The Consumers' Association.

Charng, H.-W., Piliavin, J.A. and Callero, P.L. (1988), 'Role identity and reasoned action in the prediction of repeated behavior', *Social Psychology Quarterly*, 51, 4, pp. 303-317.

Dan-Cohen, M. (1992), 'Conceptions of choice and conceptions of autonomy', *Ethics*, 102, pp. 221-243.

Davidson, A.R. and Morrison, D.M. (1983), 'Predicting contraceptive behavior from attitudes: a comparison of within- versus across-subjects procedures', *Journal of Personality and Social Psychology*, 45, pp. 997-1009.

Eagly, A.H. (1992), 'Uneven progress: social psychology and the study of attitudes', *Journal of Personality and Social Psychology*, 63, 5, pp. 693-710.

Eagly, A.H. and Chaiken, S. (1993), *The Psychology of Attitudes*, Harcourt, Brace and Jovanovich, New York.

Evans, R.I. (1988), 'Health promotion — science or ideology?', *Health Psychology*, 7 (3), pp. 203-219.

Fischhoff, B., Goitein, B. and Shapira, Z. (1982), 'The experienced utility of expected utility approaches', in Feather, N.T. (ed.), *Expectations and Actions: Expectancy-Value Models in Psychology*, Erlbaum, Hillsdale, NJ.

Gorsuch, R.L. and Ortberg, J. (1983), 'Moral obligation and attitudes: their relation to behavioral intentions', *Journal of Personality and Social Psychology*, 44, 5, pp. 1025-1028.

Herrnstein, R.J. (1990), 'Rational choice theory: necessary but not sufficient', *American Psychologist*, 45, 3, pp. 356-367.

Hewstone, M. and Young, L. (1988), 'Expectancy-value models of attitude: measurement and combination of evaluations and beliefs', *Journal of Applied Social Psychology*, 18, 11, pp. 958-971.

Hoch, S.J. and Loewenstein, G.F. (1991), 'Time-inconsistent preferences and consumer self-control', *Journal of Consumer Research*, 17, pp. 492-507.

Lang, T., Dibb, S., Cole-Hamilton, I. and Lobstein, T. (1989), *This Food Business*, A report produced by Channel 4 Television and *New Statesman and Society*.

Leather, S. (1992), 'Less money, less choice: poverty and diet in the UK today', in National Consumer Council (ed.), *Your Food: Whose Choice?*, HMSO, London.

Liska, A. E. (1984), 'A critical examination of the causal structure of the Fishbein/Ajzen attitude-behaviour model', *Social Psychology Quarterly*, 47, pp. 621-74.

Logue, A.W. (1986), *The Psychology of Eating and Drinking*, W.H. Freeman, New York.

March, J.G. (1978), 'Bounded rationality, ambiguity, and the engineering of choice', *Bell Journal of Economics*, 9, pp. 587-608.
Murcott, A. (1988), 'Sociological and social anthropological approaches to food and eating', in Bourne, G.H. (ed.), *World Review of Nutrition and Dietetics*, 55, 1-40. Karger, Basel.
Norman, P. and Smith, L. (submitted) 'Applying the Theory of Planned Behaviour to the prediction of exercise behaviour'.
Payne, J.W., Bettman, J.R. and Johnson, E.J. (1992), 'Behavioural decision research: a constructive processing perspective', *Annual Review of Psychology*, 43, pp. 87-113.
Pill, R. and Parry, O. (1989), 'Making changes — women, food and families', *Health Education Journal*, 48, 2, pp. 51-54.
Raats, M.M. (1992), *The Role of Beliefs and Sensory Responses to Milk in Determining the Selection of Milks of Different Fat Content*, unpublished doctoral thesis, University of Reading.
Rosin, S., Tuorila, H. and Uutela, A. (1992), 'Garlic: a sensory pleasure or a social nuisance?', *Appetite*, 19, pp. 133-143.
Rutter, D.R. and Bunce, D.J. (1989), 'The Theory of Reasoned Action of Fishbein and Ajzen: a test of Towriss's amended procedure for measuring beliefs', *British Journal of Social Psychology*, 28, 1, pp. 39-46.
Sarver, V.T. Jnr (1983), 'Ajzen and Fishbein's "Theory of Reasoned Action": a critical assessment', *Journal for the Theory of Social Behaviour*, 13, pp. 155-163.
Schoemaker, P.J.H. (1982), 'The expected utility model: its variants, purposes, evidence and limitations', *Journal of Economic Literature*, 20, pp. 529-563.
Schwartz, S.H. (1978), 'Temporal instability as a moderator of the attitude-behavior relationship', *Journal of Personality and Social Psychology*, 36, 7, pp. 715-724.
Shepherd, R., Sparks, P., Bellier, S. and Raats, M. (1993), 'Attitudes and choice of flavoured milks: extensions of Fishbein and Ajzen's Theory of Reasoned Action', *Food Quality and Preference*, 3, pp. 157-164.
Sparks, P. (1993), 'Attitudes, utility and moral judgements', paper presented at the General Meeting of the EAESP, Lisbon, September 15-20, 1993.
Sparks, P. and Shepherd, R. (1992), 'Self-identity and the Theory of Planned Behavior: assessing the role of identification with "green consumerism"', *Social Psychology Quarterly*, 55, 4, pp. 388-399.
Sparks, P. and Shepherd, R. (in preparation, a), 'The moral dimension of attitudes towards genetic engineering in food production'.

Sparks, P. and Shepherd, R. (in preparation, b), 'Attitudes towards dietary change: an assessment of the Theory of Planned Behaviour and the proximal antecedents of perceived behavioural control'.
Sparks, P., Hedderley, D. and Shepherd, R. (1991), Expectancy-value models of attitudes: a note on the relationship between theory and methodology, *European Journal of Social Psychology*, 21, pp. 261-271.
Sparks, P., Hedderley, D. and Shepherd, R. (1992), 'An investigation into the relationship between perceived control, attitude variability and the consumption of two common foods', *European Journal of Social Psychology*, 22, pp. 55-71.
Sparks, P., Shepherd, R. and Frewer, L.J. (in press), 'Assessing and structuring public attitudes towards the uses of gene technology in food production: the role of perceived ethical obligation', *Basic and Applied Social Psychology*.
Sparks, P., Shepherd, R., Wieringa, N. and Zimmermanns, N. (1992), 'Barriers to healthy eating: an examination of perceived behavioural control and unrealistic optimism', paper presented at the BPS Social Psychology Section Annual Conference, University of Hertfordshire, September 15-17 1992.
Sparks, P., Shepherd, R., Wieringa, N. and Zimmermanns, N. (submitted), 'Perceived behavioural control, unrealistic optimism and dietary change: an exploratory study'.
Tuorila-Ollikainen, H., Lähteenmaki, L. and Salovaara, H. (1986), 'Attitudes, norms, intentions and hedonic responses in the selection of low salt bread in a longitudinal choice experiment', *Appetite*, 7, pp. 127-39.
White, S. and Wetherell, M. (1988), 'Fear of fat: a study of discourses concerning eating patterns and body shape', paper presented at the BPS Social Psychology Section Conference, University of Kent, September 1988.
Wilson, T.D., Dunn, D.S., Kraft, D. and Lisle, D.J. (1989), 'Introspection, attitude change, and attitude-behavior consistency: the disruptive effects of explaining why we feel the way we do', in Berkowitz, L. (ed.), *Advances in Experimental Social Psychology*, Vol. 22, Academic Press, New York.
Zanna, M.P and Rempel, J.K. (1988), 'Attitudes: a new look at an old concept', in Bar-Tal, D. and Kruglanski, A.W. (eds), *The Social Psychology of Knowledge*, Cambridge University Press, Cambridge.
Zuckerman, M. and Reis, H.T. (1978), 'Comparison of three models for predicting altruistic behavior', *Journal of Personality and Social Psychology*, 36, 5, pp. 498-510.

3 Addictive behaviours: Predictors of abstinence intentions and expectations in the Theory of Planned Behaviour

Neo K. Morojele and Geoffrey M. Stephenson

Introduction

During the past decade a considerable amount of research relating to Fishbein and Ajzen's Theory of Reasoned Action (Fishbein and Ajzen, 1975; Ajzen and Fishbein, 1980) has questioned the notion that behavioural intention is the sole immediate determinant of volitional behaviour. For example, past behaviour (e.g. Bentler and Speckart, 1979; Fredricks and Dossett, 1983; Echabe, Rovira and Garate, 1988) and attitudes (e.g. Bentler and Speckart, 1979; Bagozzi, Yi and Baumgartner, 1990) have also been shown to be direct determinants of behaviour, independently of behavioural intentions.

According to the Theory of Reasoned Action, behavioural intention is the most immediate determinant of any social behaviour but only under conditions where the behaviour in question is under volitional control and behavioural intention remains unchanged. The theory proposes that an individual's intention is determined, in turn, by his or her attitude and subjective norm regarding the performance of the behaviour. Furthermore, attitude to the behaviour is accounted for by beliefs about the outcomes of the behaviour and evaluations of those outcomes. Subjective norm is determined by perceived pressure from specified significant others to carry out the behaviour and by motivation to comply with the wishes of those significant others.

The Theory of Reasoned Action has received considerable support in the prediction of a range of social behaviours (see Ajzen, 1988; Ajzen and Fishbein, 1980, for reviews). However, as we explain below, the boundary conditions of the theory are such that it fails to account adequately for behaviours that are not fully under volitional control. In this chapter we consider the ways in which the theory has been modified in order to account for those non-volitional, non-reasoned actions. We refer specifically to Ajzen's Theory of Planned Behaviour (Ajzen, 1985, 1987, 1988) and to Warshaw and Davis' approach (Warshaw and Davis, 1985), in which a distinction is made between behavioural expectation and behavioural intention. These modifications are particularly pertinent to addictive behaviours and to attempts to control them, where there is a strongly non-volitional, non-rational element. It is proposed that Ajzen's Theory of Planned Behaviour is more appropriate for the prediction of addictive behaviours than is the Theory of Reasoned Action, and furthermore that behavioural expectation is a required construct within Ajzen's framework, as the most immediate predictor of behavioural performance.

The Theory of Planned Behaviour

Icek Ajzen (Ajzen, 1985, 1988; Ajzen and Madden, 1986) extended the Theory of Reasoned Action to account for behaviours that are not fully under volitional control and introduced the Theory of Planned Behaviour. As we have seen already in this volume, the Theory of Planned Behaviour incorporates the original components of the reasoned action model, but also includes a perceived behavioural control variable, defined as 'the perceived ease or difficulty of performing the behavior' (Ajzen, 1987, p. 44). According to Ajzen (1985), where a behaviour is not fully under volitional control, perceived behavioural control and behavioural intention will together account for it, at least when perceptions of control are true reflections of actual control. The Theory of Planned Behaviour also proposes that, along with attitude and subjective norm, perceived behavioural control is a determinant of behavioural intention.

To date, support for the Theory of Planned Behaviour has come from several behavioural domains (see Ajzen, 1991, for a review). With regard to the prediction of behavioural intention, Ajzen's (1991) review showed that perceived behavioural control was a significant predictor of behavioural intention in all of 16 studies. However, the results of other studies (e.g. Fishbein and Stasson, 1990; Hinsz and Nelson, 1990; and Schlegel et al., 1992, amongst a problem drinker sample) have failed to show such an effect. Ajzen's review also revealed that, in most although not all studies, perceived behavioural control was a significant predictor of behavioural performance. Presumably, perceived behavioural control did not account for behaviours where they were largely volitional and/or involved respondents whose perceptions of control over the relevant behaviours were inaccurate. A number of additional studies that were not included in Ajzen's (1991) review have also found that, for some of their samples, there was no significant effect of perceived behavioural control on behavioural performance (e.g. DeVellis et al., 1990, on cancer screening participation amongst an average risk group; Schlegel et al., 1992, on frequency of getting drunk amongst non-problem and ex-problem drinkers; Netemeyer and Burton, 1990, on voting behaviour; Fishbein and Stasson, 1990, on attendance at telephone training sessions; Dzewaltowski, Noble and Shaw, 1990, on participation in physical activity).

Behavioural intention versus behavioural expectation

The behavioural intention-behaviour relationship has also been addressed by Warshaw and Davis (1984, 1985) in relation to behaviours that are not fully under volitional control. In particular, Warshaw and Davis (1985) noted that researchers who have applied the Theory of Reasoned Action have commonly confounded behavioural intention with a related but different construct, 'behavioural expectation'.[1] They distinguished between the two constructs by defining behavioural intention as 'the degree to which a person has formulated conscious plans to perform some specified future behavior' (1985, p. 214), in contrast with behavioural expectation, which was defined as 'the individual's estimation of the likelihood that he or she actually will perform some specified future behavior' (1985, p. 215).

Warshaw and Davis (1985) argued that intentions do not reliably account for behaviours in the case of non-volitional behaviours, outcomes or goal attainment, and/or where changes in intentions occur. They proposed that behavioural expectation is a better candidate for behavioural prediction than behavioural intention because judgements of behavioural expectation incorporate both control factors (factors that hinder or facilitate behavioural performance) and foreseeable future changes in intentions. Additionally, they considered behavioural expectations to possess self-fulfilling causal potential, partly by influencing the amount of effort the individual would be prepared to exert in his or her attempt to carry out a particular behaviour. Consequently, for behaviours that are under complete volitional control, for which control considerations are not relevant, behavioural intention may arguably remain the appropriate antecedent of behavioural performance.

The potential role of behavioural expectation in the Theory of Planned Behaviour

Close examination of Ajzen's original formulation of the Theory of Planned Behaviour reveals that he incorporated a behavioural expectation component into the model and viewed its role in a manner similar to that that seems to be implied by Warshaw and Davis (1985). Ajzen proposed that, in general, 'people will expect to perform a behavior if they intend to try it ... and if they believe (have a high subjective probability) that they can control it ...' (1985, p. 33). 'Behavioral intentions and expectations will tend to differ whenever respondents anticipate that their intentions might change or when they believe that attainment of their behavioural goal is not completely under their volitional control' (1985, p. 33). Unlike Warshaw and Davis (1985), however, Ajzen did not regard behavioural expectations as having a causal effect on actual behaviour.

The behavioural expectation variable is not mentioned in Ajzen's more recent publications on the Theory of Planned Behaviour (Ajzen and Madden, 1986; Schifter and Ajzen, 1985; Ajzen, 1987; 1988; 1991). The reasons are unclear, but probably relate to the fact that Ajzen originally referred to the prediction of behavioural goals and attempts to perform behaviours (Ajzen, 1985), but later abandoned that tack once it became evident from later applications (Schifter and Ajzen, 1985; Ajzen and Madden, 1986) that the prediction of actual behaviour was not different from the prediction of attempted behaviour.

The envisaged role and location of behavioural expectation within the Theory of Planned Behaviour is worth examining in some detail, and there are a number of reasons. First, it is clear that behavioural expectation is central to the prediction of social behaviours since it has been shown to out-predict behavioural intention in certain circumstances (Warshaw and Davis, 1984; 1985), although others have found the reverse effect (Fishbein and Stasson, 1990; Netemeyer and Burton, 1990). Second, behavioural expectation has been shown on numerous occasions (inadvertently, by researchers who have operationalized behavioural intentions as expectations) to account for actual behaviour. Third, it has been proposed by Ajzen (1985) and by Warshaw and Davis (1985) that behavioural expectation encompasses considerations of control and foreseeable changes in behavioural intention, which are some of the very factors that weaken the intention-behaviour relationship. Finally, like the Theory of Planned Behaviour, behavioural expectation is particularly relevant to the prediction of non-volitional behaviours, goals, or outcomes (Fishbein and Stasson, 1990; Sheppard, Hartwick and Warshaw, 1988). In summary, then, we are proposing that (a) behavioural expectations can be incorporated into the planned behaviour framework as a more plausible basis for prediction than behavioural intentions, especially where non-volitional behaviours, outcomes and goals are concerned; (b) perceived behavioural control and behavioural intention will bear directly on behavioural expectation; and (c) the greater the degree to which the behaviour is under volitional control, the stronger will be the relationship between behavioural intention and behavioural expectation.

Prediction of addictive behaviours

> An addiction is essentially a repetitive behaviour which is subject to powerful motivational forces. The behaviour persists in the face of societal sanctions and/or actual or potential harm to the individual or those with whom he or she comes into contact. Mostly this involves ingesting drugs (including nicotine and alcohol), but it can also involve behaviours such as gambling. There may also be addictive components to other compulsive behaviours such as overeating. (West, 1989, p. 71)

Some of the common hallmarks of addictive behaviours, namely, that they are compulsive ('powerful motivational force'), habitual and irrational ('persist in the face of societal sanctions and/or actual or potential harm'), are apparent from the above definition. Also, it is evident from the definition that while addiction tends to be associated with the use of specific substances, such as drugs and alcohol, and/or the performance of specific behaviours, such as gambling, the key feature of such behaviours is not the use of those substances or the performance of those behaviours per se, but rather, the manner (compulsively, habitually, irrationally) in which the substances are used and/or the behaviours are performed.

Addiction and the Theory of Reasoned Action To the extent that addictive behaviours are neither rational nor volitional, they are outside the range of application of the Theory of Reasoned Action. Many studies have successfully applied the Theory of Reasoned Action, or variations of it, to the prediction of intentions and performance of behaviours commonly associated with addiction, such as drinking alcoholic beverages, smoking cigarettes and marijuana, and using 'hard' drugs. The literature includes studies by Bearden and Woodside (1978), Grube, Morgan and McGree (1986), and Kilty (1978) (all of whom measured behavioural expectations rather than behavioural intentions), and others by Bentler and Speckart (1979), Budd (1986), Budd and Spencer (1984), Fishbein (1982), and Fishbein, Ajzen and McArdle (1980) (all of whom measured behavioural intention as defined by Warshaw and Davis, 1985). Other writers, including Kristiansen and Eiser (1986), and Schlegel, Crawford and Sanborn (1977) did not specify the manner in which behavioural intentions were operationalized.

It should be noted that, with the exception of the work by Fishbein, Ajzen and McArdle (1980), and Kilty (1978), all the studies were conducted amongst populations of predominantly non-'addicted' secondary school or university undergraduate students using 'addictive' substances. Fishbein,

Ajzen and McArdle's (1980) respondents were alcoholic patients, but the target behaviour in their study was not addictive behaviour but rather signing up for an alcohol treatment unit. Kilty's (1978) study included male inmates in a 'state correctional institution', all of whom were also members of Alcoholics Anonymous (although the authors note that membership did not necessarily mean that the participant had a problem with alcohol). Kilty showed that the variables of the Theory of Reasoned Action were successful in predicting drinking intentions but not drinking behaviour.

Cigarette smoking among adolescents is rather a different behaviour (from the use of alcohol and most other drugs) in that it is more likely to have been addictive among the respondents in the studies in question. Adolescent smokers smoke cigarettes more regularly than they drink alcohol and use other drugs; nicotine is considered to be more addictive than other drugs; and more adolescent tobacco users than alcohol users say they are dependent (Henningfield, Cohen and Slade, 1991). In the studies of cigarette smoking amongst undergraduate and high school students, the reasoned action model has proved successful in predicting intentions to smoke cigarettes (Budd, 1986; Grube, Morgan and McGree, 1986) and intentions to try cigarettes, start smoking, quit smoking, and change brand of cigarette (Fishbein, 1982). With respect to the prediction of cigarette *smoking* there has been some reported success for the Theory of Reasoned Action (e.g. Budd, 1986; Fishbein, 1982; Grube, Morgan and McGree, 1986), though quitting smoking has not been predicted successfully (Fishbein, 1982).

In the light of this brief review, then, there is still a need for research to examine the appropriateness of the Theory of Reasoned Action in the prediction of addictive behaviours. However, given that addictive behaviours are not fully under volitional control, the Theory of Planned Behaviour would seem to be the more appropriate model.

Addiction and the Theory of Planned Behaviour To the best of our knowledge, the only applications of the Theory of Planned Behaviour to addictive behaviours have so far been in studies conducted by Schlegel et al. (1992) and Godin et al. (1992). Schlegel et al. found that, for their non-problem drinker and ex-problem drinker samples, along with attitude and subjective norm perceived behavioural control was a significant predictor of 'intention' to get drunk but did not account for actual behaviour. Among a problem drinker group in their sample, however, perceived behavioural control (along with 'intention') was a significant predictor of behaviour but failed to account for behavioural 'intention'. Godin et al.'s (1992) study provided support for the Theory of Planned Behaviour in the prediction of both intention not to smoke cigarettes and not smoking itself for a sample of adult smokers from the general population and a sample of pregnant women. It should be noted that both Schlegel et al. and Godin et al. operationalized behavioural intention as a self-prediction or expectation. The Theory of Planned Behaviour, especially when compared with the Theory of Reasoned Action in the domain of addictive behaviours, thus remains well worth examining.

Addiction and the distinction between behavioural expectation and behavioural intention To the extent that addictive behaviours are not fully under volitional control, the distinction between behavioural expectation and intention is clearly applicable, be it in the initiation, maintenance or termination of the behaviour. Consider the 'addicted', 'heavy' smoker, for example, whose plans (intentions) to give up smoking repeatedly fail to translate into behaviour. No doubt the individual's behaviour could be predicted more reliably from his of her expectation that (s)he really will give up than from consideration of his or her plans to do so. In contrast, for the more 'occasional', 'non-addicted' smoker, plans to quit smoking altogether are more likely to translate into actually giving up — assuming that this individual's compulsion to smoke is less than in the case of the heavy smoker and that perceived control over giving up is greater, so that both reflect more closely his or her expectations about giving up.

In an application of the Theory of Reasoned Action, Fishbein (1982) found that intentions to smoke cigarettes were related to smoking behaviour for a sample of young women, whilst no such relationship was found between intentions to *quit* smoking and actual quitting for a similar group of women. He argued that the latter finding resulted from a failure to consider alternative intentions in the prediction of quitting behaviour (see Fishbein, 1982, for a more detailed discussion of this line of argument). A different explanation, however, is that smoking behaviour was under greater volitional control for the sample of young women than was *quitting* behaviour, and perhaps 'quitting expectations' would have accounted for subsequent quitting more reliably than would quitting plans.

Studies from the addiction literature have shown that people's expectations regarding whether they will be successful in abstaining or giving up various addictive substances or addictive behaviours do relate to their future behaviour (e.g. Adamson, Fostakowsky and Chebib, 1974; Gossop et al., 1990; Hall and Havassy, 1983; Howden Chapman and Huygens, 1988). The association occurs even as long as 18 months after the time of the initial measurement of the expectations (Howden Chapman and Huygens, 1988). None of the studies was conducted within Ajzen or Fishbein-Ajzen theoretical frameworks, but all of them were conducted amongst people in treatment for addictions, for whom reducing or quitting addictive behaviour of one kind or another was presumably not under volitional control.

Behavioural expectation, then, is a relevant construct for addictive behaviours. Its incorporation within Ajzen's theoretical framework, which is concerned specifically with behaviours that are not fully under volitional control, would seem to be worth examining.

The Promis Recovery Centre

The participants in the present study were individuals (referred to as patients) who were in treatment at the Promis Recovery Centre — an addiction treatment programme for alcohol, drugs and eating disorders. The Promis Recovery Centre is a residential treatment centre in Kent in the United Kingdom. The programme is based on the Minnesota Model (Cook, 1988), which in turn follows the principles of the Anonymous Fellowship groups, of which Alcoholics Anonymous is probably the best known. One of the key tenets of the treatment philosophy is that the attainment of abstinence (a goal of treatment) is the individual's personal responsibility. The main role of treatment is to introduce and make available to the patients methods by which they can bring about abstinence. During treatment the patients work through the first five of the Anonymous Fellowships' twelve steps. The treatment lasts for six to twelve weeks.

Aims of the study

The target behavioural outcome in the present study is abstinence and/or sensible eating, which are some of the main goals of treatment. The aims of the study were: (i) To compare the utility of the Theories of Reasoned Action and Planned Behaviour in the prediction of abstinence intentions. It is predicted that the Theory of Planned Behaviour will be superior to the Theory of Reasoned Action in the prediction of abstinence intentions. In addition, it is predicted that the models will be more successful in the prediction of abstinence intentions than abstinence expectations. (ii) To determine the role of behavioural expectation within the framework of the Theory of Planned Behaviour. It is proposed that abstinence expectations are based on abstinence related intention, perceived control, and an interaction between intention and perceived control. Furthermore, we predict that the effect of attitude, subjective norm, and perceived behavioural control on behavioural expectation will be mediated by behavioural intention.

Method

Participants

The participants were divided into two sub-samples: (i) Intake Sample — The intake sample was made up of 87 patients who completed the questionnaire and also completed treatment. There were 59 women and 28 men, ranging in age from 16 to 67 years. The mean was 32 years. (ii) Discharge Sample — The discharge sample was a sub-sample of the intake sample and comprised 61 patients who completed questionnaires on discharge, and also completed treatment. Mean age (32 years) and sex distribution (41 women and 20 men) were similar to those of the intake sample. The mean duration of treatment for the patients was 67.2 days (s.d. = 18.5). Further details about the sample are given in Morojele and Stephenson (1992).

Measures and procedure

A self-report questionnaire was employed, consisting of items making up measures of intention, expectation, and global and belief based measures of attitude, subjective norm, and perceived behavioural control with respect to sensible eating/abstinence from alcohol and drugs in the future. The belief based measures of attitude, subjective norm, and perceived control, however, are not the focus of the present report and will not be discussed. The respondents were informed that they were to answer the questions in terms of their relevant disorder/primary drug of choice, and that the 'future' referred to 'from now onward'.

A measure of 'attitude' to future abstinence/sensible eating was made up of 6 items. The respondents indicated the extent to which their future abstinence/sensible eating was likely to be 'good-bad', 'rewarding-punishing', 'desirable-undesirable', 'wise-foolish', 'beneficial-harmful', and 'positive-negative', on seven point bipolar scales. The measure of attitude yielded a Cronbach's alpha of 0.82 on intake and 0.72 on discharge. For a measure of 'subjective norm', the participants indicated on a seven point scale the likelihood that 'most people who are important to me think I should abstain/eat sensibly in the future'. Four items made up a measure of perceived behavioural control: 'For me to eat sensibly/abstain totally in the future would be easy-difficult', 'Nothing could prevent me from eating sensibly/abstaining totally from alcohol/drugs if I wanted to', 'My accomplishment of sensible eating/total abstinence from alcohol/drugs in the future is entirely up to me', and 'If I wanted to, I could eat sensibly/

abstain totally from alcohol/drugs in the future'. Cronbach's alpha for this measure was 0.43 on intake and 0.44 on discharge. Finally, the items 'I intend to eat sensibly/abstain totally from alcohol/drugs in the future', and 'I expect to eat sensibly/abstain totally from alcohol/drugs in the future' were measures of abstinence intentions and abstinence expectations respectively.

The study employed a repeated measures design, in that the patients completed the questionnaires on admission (during their first two weeks in treatment, approximately), and again on discharge from treatment (during their final week). The patients were informed that their responses would be confidential.

Results

Multiple regression analyses were conducted in order (i) to compare the utility of the Theories of Reasoned Action and Planned Behaviour, using both abstinence intention and abstinence expectation as criterion variables; (ii) to examine whether behavioural intention mediates effects on expectation of attitude, subjective norm, and perceived control; and, (iii) to test the prediction that the most direct determinants of abstinence expectation are intention, perceived control, and an interaction between intention and perceived control. The respondents' intake and discharge results are presented separately.

Results on admission

Comparing the Theories of Reasoned Action and Planned Behaviour Table 3.1 presents the correlations between the variables in the models. Hierarchical multiple regression analyses were conducted to compare the relative powers of the models of reasoned action and planned behaviour in the prediction of abstinence intention. Attitude and subjective norm were entered on the first step, and perceived control was entered on the second step. The results are presented in the upper half of Table 3.2. Subjective norm relating to abstinence was a significant predictor of abstinence intentions, whereas the effect of attitude on intention was only marginally significant. The inclusion of perceived control in the second step did not increase the predictive power of the model. The Theory of Planned Behaviour was therefore no more successful than the Theory of Reasoned Action in predicting abstinence intentions.

To determine whether abstinence expectation could be considered an appropriate substitute for abstinence intention, a second hierarchical

Table 3.1
Admission: Correlations between attitude, subjective norm, perceived control, intention, and expectation relating to abstinence

	Attitude	Subjective Norm	Perceived Control	Intention
Attitude	—			
Subjective Norm	0.30**	—	—	—
Perceived Control	0.05	0.32**	—	—
Intention	0.28*	0.34**	0.13	—
Expectation	0.26*	0.29**	0.10	0.33**

* $p < 0.05$ ** $p < 0.01$

Table 3.2
Admission: Hierarchical regression coefficients. Prediction of intention and expectation from attitude, subjective norm, and perceived control

	Beta	F (model)	df	R^2
Prediction of intention				
Step 1: Theory of Reasoned Action				
Attitude	0.20†	6.69**	2,75	0.15**
Subjective Norm	0.28*	—	—	—
Step 2: Theory of Planned Behaviour				
Attitude	0.20†	4.44**	3,74	0.15**
Subjective Norm	0.27*	—	—	—
Perceived Control	0.04	—	—	—
Prediction of expectation				
Step 1: Theory of Reasoned Action				
Attitude	0.19	4.80*	2,75	0.11*
Subjective Norm	0.23*	—	—	—
Step 2: Theory of Planned Behaviour				
Attitude	0.19	3.17*	3,74	0.11*
Subjective Norm	0.22†	—	—	—
Perceived Control	0.02	—	—	—

Note: To take into account the negatively skewed distributions of scores for attitude, subjective norm, intention and expectation, the variables were reflected and then inversely transformed.

† $p < 0.10$ * $p < 0.05$ ** $p < 0.01$

multiple regression analysis was conducted, using expectation as the criterion variable. The results are presented in the lower half of Table 3.2. In the first step, subjective norm was the only significant predictor. The inclusion of perceived behavioural control in the second step did not significantly increase the predictive power of the model.

Predictors of abstinence expectation The results presented so far have provided some support for the Theory of Reasoned Action in the prediction of both intention and expectation. As expected, subjective norm was found to be a better predictor of abstinence intention ($R^2 = 0.15$) than abstinence expectation ($R^2 = 0.11$), although the difference was not large. To determine whether the effect of subjective norm on expectation was mediated by intention, a multiple regression analysis was performed in which expectation was regressed on attitude, subjective norm, and perceived control, as before, and intention was included as an additional variable. It was assumed that the significant effect of subjective norm on expectation would become non-significant (with the inclusion of intention) if the effect of subjective norm on expectation was mediated by intention. As shown in Table 3.3, with the inclusion of intention in the equation the effect of subjective norm on expectation ceased to be statistically significant. Moreover, the predictive power of the model was significantly greater ($R^2 = 0.16$) when intention was included than when it was not ($R^2 = 0.11$; F-change = 4.01, df = 1,73; $p < 0.05$). This result supports our prediction that the effect of subjective norm on expectation is mediated by intention.

To test the hypothesis that expectation is based on perceived control, intention, and an interaction between intention and perceived control, a further hierarchical multiple regression analysis was conducted. On the first step of the analysis, expectation was regressed on intention and perceived control, and the interaction term was included in the analysis on the second step. The results are presented in Table 3.4, from which it can be seen that on the first step only intention was a significant predictor of expectation. The addition of the interaction term on the second step did not increase predictive validity.

Results on discharge

Comparing the Theories of Reasoned Action and Planned Behaviour Table 3.5 presents the correlations between the variables in the models. Hierarchical multiple regression analyses were conducted to compare the Theory of Reasoned Action and the Theory of Planned Behaviour in the prediction of abstinence intention. As can be seen from the upper half of

Table 3.3
Admission: Multiple regression coefficients. Prediction of expectation from attitude, subjective norm, perceived control, and intention

	Beta	F (model)	df	R^2
Attitude	0.14	3.48*	4,73	0.16*
Subjective Norm	0.16	—	—	—
Perceived Control	0.01	—	—	—
Intention	0.23*			

* $p < 0.05$

Table 3.4
Admission: Hierarchical regression and correlation coefficients. Prediction of expectation from intention, perceived control, and intention x perceived control

	r	Beta	F (model)	df	R^2
Step 1					
Perceived Control	0.10	0.06	4.72*	2,75	0.11*
Intention	0.33**	0.32**	—	—	—
Step 2					
Perceived Control	0.10	–0.27	3.53*	3,74	0.13*
Intention	0.33**	0.32**	—	—	—
Intention x Perceived Control	0.14	0.35	—	—	—

* $p < 0.05$ ** $p < 0.01$

Table 3.5
Discharge: Correlations between attitude, subjective norm, perceived control, intention, and expectation relating to abstinence

	Attitude	Subjective Norm	Perceived Control	Intention
Attitude	—			
Subjective Norm	0.32*	—	—	—
Perceived Control	0.11	0.18	—	—
Intention	–0.10	0.05	0.04	—
Expectation	0.07	0.19	0.33*	0.50***

* $p < 0.05$ *** $p < 0.001$

Table 3.6, none of the variation was explained by attitude or subjective norm. Furthermore, perceived control added nothing. In other words, there was no support for the utility of either the Theory of Reasoned Action or the Theory of Planned Behaviour in the prediction of abstinence intention on discharge. Hierarchical regression analyses were then performed to compare the predictive powers of the two theories in the prediction of abstinence *expectation* on discharge. Neither subjective norm nor attitude was a significant predictor on the first step of the analysis (lower half of Table 3.6). The addition of perceived control to the equation on the second step led to an increase in R^2 to 0.12 ($df = 3,55$, $F = 2.61$, $p = 0.06$).

Predictors of abstinence expectation Since it was found on discharge that attitude, subjective norm, and perceived control accounted for none of the variation in intention, the effects of the predictor variables on expectation could not be mediated by intention. Also, as is apparent from Table 3.6, only perceived control had a direct effect on expectation. By using hierarchical multiple regression analyses once more, we tested the prediction that abstinence expectations were explained by intention and perceived control, and additionally by an interaction between them. Intention and perceived control were entered together on the first step, followed by the interaction term on the second step. Intention and perceived control were both significant predictors of abstinence expectation (Table 3.7). Furthermore, the inclusion of the interaction term yielded a significant increase in R^2 from 0.35 to 0.40 (F-change = 4.11, $df = 1,54$, $p < 0.05$). This result supports the prediction that perceived control, intention, and an interaction between perceived control and intention are significant predictors of abstinence expectation on discharge.

Discussion

One of our main arguments in this chapter has been that the Theory of Reasoned Action is not appropriate for the prediction of behavioural outcomes or goals associated with addiction, given that addictive behaviours tend to be of a 'compulsive', non-'rational', and relatively non-volitional nature. Very few applications of the theory have been successful in the prediction of addictive behaviours. We have further argued that Ajzen's extension of the theory to the Theory of Planned Behaviour, and Warshaw and Davis' discussion of behavioural expectation as a more plausible antecedent of behavioural performance than behavioural

Table 3.6
Discharge: Hierarchical regression coefficients. Prediction of intention and expectation from attitude, subjective norm, and perceived control

	Beta	F (model)	df	R^2
Prediction of intention				
Step 1: Theory of Reasoned Action				
Attitude	–0.13	0.48	2,56	0.02
Subjective Norm	0.09	—	—	—
Step 2: Theory of Planned Behaviour				
Attitude	–0.13	0.33	3,55	0.02
Subjective Norm	0.08	—	—	—
Perceived Control	0.03	—	—	—
Prediction of expectation				
Step 1: Theory of Reasoned Action				
Attitude	0.00	1.02	2,56	0.04
Subjective Norm	0.19	—	—	—
Step 2: Theory of Planned Behaviour				
Attitude	0.01	2.61†	3,55	0.12†
Subjective Norm	0.13	—	—	—
Perceived Control	0.30*	—	—	—

† $p < 0.10$ * $p < 0.05$

Table 3.7
Discharge: Hierarchical regression and correlation coefficients. Prediction of expectation from intention, perceived control, and intention x perceived control

	r	Beta	F (model)	df	R^2
Step 1					
Perceived Control	0.50***	0.49***	14.77***	2,55	0.35***
Intention	0.33*	0.31**	—	—	—
Step 2					
Intention	0.50***	0.70***	11.78***	3,54	0.40***
Perceived Control	0.33*	0.96**	—	—	—
Intention x Perceived Control	0.38**	–0.72*	—	—	—

* $p < 0.05$ ** $p < 0.01$ *** $p < 0.001$

intention, were pertinent for addictive behaviours and outcomes. With long term outcome (abstinence) data unavailable, our analyses have focused on the prediction of abstinence intention. It was expected that (i) the Theory of Planned Behaviour would be superior to the Theory of Reasoned Action in the prediction of abstinence intentions; (ii) any effects of attitude and subjective norm on expectation would be mediated by intention; (iii) perceived control would have both a direct and an indirect effect (mediated by intention) on expectation; and (iv) expectation would be based on intention, perceived control, and an interaction between intention and perceived control. The findings support some but not all of our predictions.

Comparison of the Theories of Reasoned Action and Planned Behaviour

Contrary to our expectations, the results failed to provide support for the superiority of the Theory of Planned Behaviour over the Theory of Reasoned Action in the prediction of abstinence intentions. Perceived control bore no relation to intention either on intake or on discharge. These results are somewhat surprising given that the Theory of Planned Behaviour was developed precisely to account for behaviours that are not fully under volitional control, and also given that most, though not all, studies that have applied the Theory of Planned Behaviour have found that perceived control is a significant predictor of behavioural intention. This raises the question of whether there are conditions under which perceived control may have no bearing on intention. Ajzen (1988) proposes that people are not likely to form strong intentions to perform behaviours when they believe they lack the necessary resources and opportunities to perform them. With regard to the quitting of addictive behaviours, however, it would seem that 'addicted' people commonly have strong intentions to abstain/quit, *even though* they believe they do not have the necessary willpower, resources, or facilitative conditions for their goal to be attained.

It is significant that on arrival at the treatment centre the respondents' plans to attain their goal of abstinence were based on their subjective norm – presumably because important others had expressed a need for them to do something about their addiction, which was the main reason why they too intended to recover and had entered treatment. It is interesting that on discharge the respondents' intentions could not be explained by their attitude, subjective norms, or perceived control relating to abstinence. When the respondents' abstinence *expectations* were considered as a substitute for abstinence intention, it emerged that on admission they were based only on subjective norm, but that subjective norm had an indirect effect which was mediated by intention. On discharge, in comparing the Theories of Reasoned Action and Planned Behaviour using expectation in place of intention, only perceived control was a significant predictor of expectation, and its effect was not this time mediated by intention.

In summary, we have found no evidence that the Theory of Planned Behaviour is superior to the Theory of Reasoned Action in predicting intentions to eat sensibly/abstain totally from alcohol and/or drugs amongst the patients in the treatment centre. The Theory of Reasoned Action was shown to be useful in the prediction of abstinence intention with subjective norm as the sole predictor, but subjective norm explained only a small proportion of the variance. When expectation was used as a substitute for intention the effect of subjective norm was found to be mediated by intention. On discharge, abstinence expectation proved to be a poor substitute for intention, since neither attitude nor subjective norm accounted for it, and only perceived control explained any of the variance. We infer from these results that expectation plays a distinct and important role in the Fishbein-Ajzen and Ajzen explanatory frameworks.

The role of expectation

Following the analyses of Warshaw and Davis (1985) and Ajzen (1985) in his original formulation of the Theory of Planned Behaviour, our aim was to determine the extent to which expectation could be explained. Specifically, it was predicted that intention, perceived control, and an interaction between behavioural intention and perceived control would be the most immediate antecedents of expectation. The discharge results provided support for both predictions, for not only did perceived control and intentions account for expectations but so did the interaction between the two variables. On admission to treatment, however, only behavioural intention was a significant predictor: perceived control and the interaction between perceived control and intention were not.

These last findings suggest that there were different factors bearing on admission expectations and discharge expectations. One explanation may relate to the emphasis of the treatment philosophy on personal responsibility for recovery. Previous data from the same sample of patients (Morojele and Stephenson, 1992) have revealed that there was a dramatic increase in patients' perceived control relating to abstinence between admission and discharge. On entry to treatment respondents were less inclined to attribute responsibility for their abstinence (recovery) to themselves, and consequently were less inclined to base their self-predictions of future abstinence on their own efforts and/or ability. By the end of treatment, when perceptions of control were considerably increased, those perceptions had a clear bearing on expectations. Our results also support the prediction that the relationship between intention and expectation is a function of the degree to which behaviour is, or is perceived to be, under volitional control. Although this was the case for respondents' results on discharge, however, no such effect was observed on admission. In conclusion, our findings thus point to the need for: (1) further extensions to the Theories of Reasoned Action and Planned Behaviour so that addictive behaviours can be better explained; (2) the inclusion of behavioural expectation in any such extension; and (3) further examination of the relative importance of expectation and intention.

Acknowledgements

The research reported in this chapter was part of the first author's PhD work and was funded by the Promis Trust. We are grateful to Dr Robert Lefever and to the staff members and patients of the Promis Recovery Centre for their cooperation. We are also grateful to those who commented on a previous draft of the report, and to Dr Derek Rutter for his support.

Notes

1. Examination of applications of the Theory of Planned Behaviour also reveals that a number of researchers have operationalized intention as a self-prediction or behavioural expectation (e.g. Beck and Ajzen, 1991; DeVellis et al., 1990; Dzewaltowski, Noble and Shaw, 1990; Godin et al. 1992; Hinsz and Nelson, 1990; Parker et al. 1992; Schlegel et al. 1992).

References

Adamson, J.D., Fostakowsky, R.T. and Chebib, F.S. (1974), 'Measures associated with outcome on one year follow-up of male alcoholics', *British Journal of Addiction*, 69, pp. 325-335.

Ajzen, I. (1985), 'From intentions to actions: a theory of planned behavior', in Kuhl, J. and Beckman, J. (eds), *Action-Control: From Cognition to Behavior*, Springer, Heidelberg, pp. 11-39.

Ajzen, I. (1987), 'Attitudes, traits, and actions: dispositional prediction of behavior in personality and social psychology', in Berkowitz, L. (ed.), *Advances in Experimental Social Psychology*, Vol. 20, Academic Press, New York, pp. 1-63.

Ajzen, I. (1988), *Attitudes, Personality and Behaviour*, Milton Keynes, Open University Press.

Ajzen, I. (1991), 'The Theory of Planned Behavior', *Organizational Behavior and Human Decision Processes*, 50, pp. 179-211.

Ajzen, I. and Fishbein, M. (1980), *Understanding Attitudes and Predicting Social Behavior*, Prentice Hall, Englewood Cliffs, NJ.

Ajzen, I. and Madden, T.J. (1986), 'Prediction of goal-directed behavior: attitudes, intentions and perceived behavioral control', *Journal of Experimental Social Psychology*, 22, pp. 453-474.

Bagozzi, R.P., Yi, Y. and Baumgartner, J. (1990), 'The level of effort required for behavior as a moderator of the attitude-behavior relation', *European Journal of Social Psychology*, 20, pp. 45-59.

Bearden, W.O and Woodside, A.G. (1978), 'Situational and extended attitude models as predictors of marijuana intentions and reported behavior', *Journal of Social Psychology*, 106, pp. 57-67.

Beck, L., and Ajzen, I. (1991), 'Predicting dishonest actions using the Theory of Planned Behavior', *Journal of Research in Personality*, 25, pp. 285-301.

Bentler, P.M., and Speckart, G. (1979), 'Models of attitude-behavior relations', *Psychological Review*, 86, pp. 452-464.

Budd, R.J. (1986), 'Cigarette use: the need to incorporate measures of salience in the Theory of Reasoned Action', *Journal of Applied Social Psychology*, 16 (8), pp. 663-685.

Budd, R.J. and Spencer, C.P. (1984), 'Predicting undergraduates' intentions to drink', *Journal of Studies on Alcohol*, 45 (2), pp. 179-183.

Cook, C.C.H. (1988), 'The Minnesota Model in the management of drug and alcohol dependency: miracle, method or myth? Part I. Philosophy and the programme', *British Journal of Addiction*, 83, pp. 735-748.

DeVellis, B.M., Blalock, S.J. and Sandler, R.S. (1990), 'Predicting participation in cancer screening: the role of perceived behavioral control', *Journal of Applied Social Psychology*, 20 (8), pp. 639-660.

Dzewaltowski, D.A., Noble, J.M. and Shaw, J.M. (1990), 'Physical activity participation: social cognitive theory versus the Theories of Reasoned Action and Planned Behavior', *Journal of Sport and Exercise Psychology*, 12, pp. 388-405.

Echabe, A.E., Rovira, D.P. and Garate, J.F.V. (1988), 'Testing Ajzen and Fishbein's attitudes model: the prediction of voting', *European Journal of Social Psychology*, 18, pp. 181-189.

Fishbein, M. (1982), 'Social psychological analysis of smoking behaviour', in Eiser, J.R. (ed.), *Social Psychology and Behavioural Medicine*, John Wiley, Chichester, pp. 179-197.

Fishbein, M. and Ajzen, I. (1975), *Belief, Attitude, Intention, and Behavior: An Introduction to Theory and Research*, Addison-Wesley, Reading, MA.

Fishbein, M., Ajzen, I. and McArdle, J. (1980), 'Changing the behavior of alcoholics: effects of persuasive communication', in Ajzen, I. and Fishbein, M. (eds), *Understanding Attitudes and Predicting Social Behavior*, Prentice-Hall, Englewood Cliffs, NJ, pp. 196-216.

Fishbein, M and Stasson, M. (1990), 'The role of desires, self-prediction, and perceived control in the prediction of training session attendance', *Journal of Applied Social Psychology*, 20 (3), pp. 173-198.

Fredricks, A.J. and Dossett, D.L. (1983), 'Attitude-behavior relations: a comparison of the Fishbein-Ajzen and the Bentler-Speckart models', *Journal of Personality and Social Psychology*, 45, pp. 501-512.

Godin, G., Valois, P., Lepage, L. and Desharnais, R. (1992), 'Predictors of smoking behaviour. An application of Ajzen's Theory of Planned Behaviour', *British Journal of Addiction*, 87 (9), pp. 1335-1343.

Gossop, M., Green, L., Phillips, G. and Bradley, B. (1990), 'Factors predicting outcome among opiate addicts after treatment', *British Journal of Clinical Psychology*, 29, pp. 209-216.

Grube, J.W., Morgan, M. and McGree, S.T. (1986), 'Attitudes and normative beliefs as predictors of smoking intentions and behaviors: a test of three models', *British Journal of Social Psychology*, 25, pp. 81-93.

Hall, S. and Havassy, B. (1983), 'Commitment to abstinence and relapse to tobacco, alcohol and opiates', in Tims, F. and Leukefeld, C. (eds), *Relapse and Recovery in Drug Abuse*, NIDA Research Monograph, 72, pp. 108-35.

Henningfield, J.E., Cohen, C. and Slade, J.D. (1991), 'Is nicotine more addictive than cocaine?', *British Journal of Addiction*, 86 (5), pp. 565-569.

Hinsz, V.B. and Nelson, L.C. (1990), 'Testing models of turnover intentions with University Faculty', *Journal of Applied Social Psychology*, 20 (1), pp. 68-84.

Howden Chapman, P.L. and Huygens, I. (1988), 'An evaluation of three treatment programmes for alcoholism: an experimental study with 6- and 18-month follow-ups', *British Journal of Addiction*, 83, pp. 67-81.

Kilty, K.M. (1978), 'Attitudinal and normative variables as predictors of drinking behavior', *Journal of Studies on Alcohol*, 39 (7), pp. 1178-1194.

Kristiansen, C.M. and Eiser, J.R. (1986), 'Predicting health-related intentions from attitudes and normative beliefs: the role of health locus of control', *British Journal of Social Psychology*, 25, pp. 67-70.

Morojele, N.K. and Stephenson, G.M. (1992), 'The Minnesota Model in the treatment of addictions: a social psychological assessment of changes in beliefs and attributions', *Journal of Community and Applied Social Psychology*, 2 (1), pp. 25-41.

Netemeyer, R.G. and Burton, S. (1990), Examining the relationship between voting behavior, intention, perceived behavioral control, and expectation, *Journal of Applied Social Psychology*, 29 (8), pp. 661-680.

Parker, D., Manstead, A.S.R., Stradling, S.G., Reason, J.T. and Baxter, J.S. (1992), 'Intention to commit driving violations: an application of the Theory of Planned Behaviour', *Journal of Applied Psychology*, 77 (1), pp. 94-101.

Schifter, D. B. and Ajzen, I. (1985), 'Intention, perceived control, and weight loss: an application of the Theory of Planned Behaviour', *Journal of Personality and Social Psychology*, 49, pp. 843-851.

Schlegel, R.P., Crawford, C.A. and Sanborn, M.D. (1977), 'Correspondence and mediational properties of the Fishbein Model: an application to adolescent alcohol use', *Journal of Experimental Social Psychology*, 13, pp. 421-430.

Schlegel, R.P., D'Avernas, J.R., Zanna, M.P., DeCourville, N.H. and Manske, S.R. (1992), 'Problem drinking: a problem for the Theory of Reasoned Action?', *Journal of Applied Social Psychology*, 22 (5), pp. 358-385.

Sheppard, B.H., Hartwick, J. and Warshaw, P.R. (1988), 'The Theory of Reasoned Action: a meta-analysis of past research with recommendations for modifications and future research', *Journal of Consumer Research*, 15, pp. 325-343.

Warshaw, P.R. and Davis, F.D. (1984), 'Self-understanding and the accuracy of behavioral expectations', *Personality and Social Psychology Bulletin*, 10, pp. 111-118.

Warshaw, P.R. and Davis, F.D. (1985), 'Disentangling behavioral intention and behavioral expectation', *Journal of Experimental Social Psychology*, 21, pp. 213-228.

West, R. (1989), 'The psychological basis of addiction', *International Review of Psychiatry*, 1 (1/2), pp. 71-80.

4 The past predicts the future: Interpreting behaviour-behaviour relationships in social psychological models of health behaviour

Stephen Sutton

Introduction

The best predictor of future behaviour is very often an earlier measure of the same behaviour. This observation is true as much for health and safety behaviours as for behaviours in other domains. In spite of this, social psychologists have persisted with the idea that concepts such as attitudes, beliefs, expectations, values, and intentions should provide a sufficient explanation of behaviour. For example, there is no place for past behaviour in the widely used Theory of Reasoned Action (Ajzen and Fishbein, 1980), or its extension, the Theory of Planned Behaviour (Ajzen, 1988, 1991). In the Theory of Reasoned Action, the person's intention to perform (or not to perform) a behaviour is held to be both the immediate determinant and the best single predictor of that behaviour. Prior behaviour is treated just like any other external variable (e.g. age, social class, neuroticism) whose effects on future behaviour are assumed to be mediated by intention. In the same way, prior behaviour can influence current intention only by influencing its theoretical determinants, namely attitude towards the behaviour and subjective norm. Other versions of the expectancy-value model make similar assumptions about the sufficiency of the model's internal variables. According to the Theory of Planned Behaviour, future behaviour may be influenced by perceived behavioural control as well as by intention. Thus prior behaviour, and other external variables, may affect future behaviour through either or both of these intervening variables but is predicted not to have a direct influence.

However, there is increasing evidence, some of which is reviewed here, that past behaviour may have independent effects on current intentions (i.e. effects not mediated by its theoretical antecedents) and, more importantly, that past behaviour frequently bypasses intention and has an independent influence on future behaviour. This chapter focuses on the second of these observations. Where such independent effects of prior behaviour on future behaviour are found, they are usually explained by brief reference to habit, learning, or reinforcement. (Indeed, we have invoked habit to explain our own findings.) The aim of this chapter is to offer a more detailed analysis of behaviour-behaviour relationships in the domain of health and safety behaviours.

Plan of the chapter

We start by discussing an abstract example using simple causal models of intention and behaviour. This is followed by a selective review of theory and research on the role of habit in determining health behaviours. We then discuss the factors that influence the size, direction, and interpretation of the behaviour-behaviour relationship and present a list of recommendations for maximizing the behaviour-behaviour correlation. Then, four examples drawn from our studies of smoking, seat belt use, and breast screening attendance are discussed in more detail. These include an example of a negative behaviour-behaviour relationship. We then make a distinction between habits and routines and suggest that many of the behaviours referred to as habits in the literature on health behaviours are more appropriately regarded as routines. We also discuss non-actions, inertia, and decision making processes that act to reduce change. Finally, we offer some suggestions for future research.

An abstract example using simple causal models

To fix ideas, consider a two wave prospective design in which measures of a given health or safety behaviour are obtained at two different time points on the same sample of subjects. We will assume for present purposes that the two measures (B1, B2) are identical. In some of the studies described later, the measures were similar but not identical. Suppose that behavioural intentions (I1) are also assessed at Time 1 and that I1 are *correspondent* with the measures of behaviour (i.e. they are measured at the same level of specificity or generality). The aim is to predict and explain variation in behaviour at Time 2.

In studies using this design, the observed correlation between B1 and B2 will typically be large and positive. In this situation, the correlation coefficient is a measure of change, or rather stability (lack of change). If all subjects retain their position relative to their neighbours, then the correlation will be perfect (or as near perfect as permitted by the range and distributions of the two measures). This would be the case, of course, even if there was a change in overall mean or absolute level. In practice, however, the observed correlation will always be less than the theoretical maximum, indicating that some change has occurred. Although the major factors underlying the behaviour may remain unchanged, there will inevitably be changes in mood, arousal, ambient light, background noise, writing implement, the speed with which the questionnaire is read, and numerous other minor influences, which result in some subjects giving a different answer on occasion 2. Subjects at the extremes of the distribution (those who have relatively high or relatively low scores at Time 1) will include some for whom these minor sources of error have happened to work in combination to pull them in that direction. When these extreme subjects are assessed again at Time 2, the chances are that the combination of minor influences will tend to be less potent. We would therefore expect that subjects with extreme scores at Time 1 will have less extreme scores at Time 2, and that their places in the distribution will be taken by other subjects who happen to experience a relatively potent combination of minor influences on occasion 2. This is the phenomenon known as *regression towards the mean*. To the extent that the aggregate effect of these random measurement errors is small, the behavioural measure has high reliability. A reliable measure is one that reflects one or more major factors and which, if these underlying factors remain unchanged over a given time period, will show little manifest change. The correlation between B1 and B2, then, is a measure of stability and — given certain assumptions and an implicit or explicit measurement model — also an index of reliability.

If we regress B2 on B1 and represent the result as a simple path diagram (B1→B2), the coefficient on this path, in standardized form, will be equal to the correlation coefficient in this simple case. Suppose that the path coefficient (beta) was 0.80. The causal interpretation is that a change of one standard deviation unit in B1 would produce a change of 0.80 standard deviation units in B2. This effect could operate either directly or through other variables. These other variables may have been measured but not included in the model (i.e. behavioural intention) or they may have been omitted from the study. Alternatively, the observed correlation between B1 and B2 may be due to one or more variables influencing behaviour at both time points, in which case the simple path diagram shown above is not an accurate representation of the underlying causal process.

So far, there are only two variables in the model (B1 and B2). If we regress B2 on B1 and I1, then, assuming that the behaviour is under volitional control (i.e. that the person can decide at will to perform or not perform the behaviour) and that intentions do not change, the Theory of

Reasoned Action would make the following predictions: (1) the effect of I1 on B2 controlling for B1 will be large and positive; and (2) the effect of B1 on B2 controlling for I1 will be zero, i.e. the B1-B2 correlation can be entirely accounted for by the correlation between B1 and I1 and the putative causal effect of I1 on B2. Now suppose the B1-B2 path is significantly different from zero. This would imply that prior behaviour circumnavigates intentions on its way to influencing subsequent behaviour. Again this effect could work directly or through other variables (excluding I1, of course, which has already been controlled for). As before, alternative interpretations in terms of omitted variables influencing both B1 and B2 (or I1 and B2) must be considered.

We made the assumption that intentions do not change, i.e. that I1 is an accurate measure not only of intentions at Time 1 but also of intentions just prior to the behaviour being performed, if indeed it was performed. To the extent that intentions do change, the lower the I1-B2 correlation and the greater the potential for other variables to predict B2. The assumption was also made that the behaviour is under volitional control. If it is not, then failure to translate intention into action will be reflected in a reduced correlation between I1 and B2. (Note that the Theory of Planned Behaviour was developed to account for behaviours that are not completely under the individual's control.)

Measurement factors may also influence the results. For example, if the measure of I1 has low reliability relative to the measures of behaviour, this would lead to the I1-B2 effect being underestimated and, to the extent that B1 and I1 are correlated (as they are likely to be), B1 will receive credit for the effect of I1; in other words, the B1-B2 path will be overestimated and the I1-B2 path underestimated. We refer to other measurement problems in a later section.

Theory and research on the role of habit in determining health behaviours

Although the concept of habit has a venerable history in the psychology of learning (e.g. Hull, 1943), social psychologists have preferred explanations in terms of attitudes and other acquired behavioural dispositions (Campbell, 1963). However, there have been one or two notable exceptions. Triandis (1977) held that the probability of an act depends on three major factors: habit, intention, and facilitating conditions. Habit is measured simply by the number of times the behaviour has previously been performed by the person, regardless of the number of times it has been reinforced. Triandis made a clear distinction between 'unexamined', overlearned, automatic (habitual) behaviour and 'carefully examined', deliberate, thoughtful, conscious (intentional) behaviour. According to Triandis, the relative importance of the two components varies depending on the kind of social behaviour being analysed. For example, behaviours used in non-verbal communication are largely under habit control; other behaviours like voting may be entirely under intentional control. In the Triandis model, habit and intention are related as follows: 'If intentions are relatively constant over time, they will cause the same behaviour over and over. Habit reflects the frequency of this behaviour. As behaviour repeatedly takes place, habit increases and becomes a better predictor of behaviour than behavioural intentions' (pp. 204-5). Triandis also states that 'when a behaviour is new, untried, and unlearned, the behavioural-intention component will be solely responsible for the behaviour, while, when the behaviour is old, well learned, or overlearned and has occurred many times before in the organism's life span, it is very likely to be under the control of the habit component' (p. 205). Of course, the first part of the statement is true simply as a consequence of the way habit is defined.

Few applications of the Triandis model have appeared in the literature to date (for a recent application of the model to exercise, see Valois, Desharnais and Godin, 1988). However, papers reporting studies in which effects of past behaviour are observed frequently refer to his work. Ronis, Yates and Kirscht (1989) have recently developed the Triandis model in the context of repeated health related behaviours. They use slightly different terminology: where Triandis talks about intentions and habits, Ronis and colleagues talk about decisions and habits, or reasoned and unreasoned influences on behaviour. They define habit as 'an action that has been done many times and has become automatic' (p. 218). They suggest that many of the special characteristics of repeated behaviours appear only if the behaviour has been repeated both frequently (at least twice a month) and extensively (at least ten times). (Note that this would exclude monthly breast self-examination, going for an annual health check, and many other repeated health actions.) In agreement with Triandis, they argue that repeated behaviours may be largely determined by habits rather than by reasoned influences, although the latter are important in the initiation and modification of habits. Ronis and colleagues recommend that, instead of using past behaviour as an index of habit, measures of habit should be developed that ask about the special characteristics of habitual or automatic behaviours, for example low level of awareness.

Although Ronis et al. assert that relatively little attention has been paid by researchers to repeated health related actions, it is worth noting that most health related behaviours are repeatable. The examples they give of non-repeated behaviours (having an influenza vaccination, having surgery, voting for fluoridation, being screened for a genetic disorder) are all in principle capable of being repeated.

In studies in this area, habit has generally been equated with past behaviour. A study by Wittenbraker, Gibbs and Kahle (1983) on seat belt use is of interest because these authors attempted to distinguish between habit and past behaviour using the framework of the Theory of Reasoned Action. They defined habit as past behaviour that is attributed by the individual to force of habit. They showed that habit at Time 1 predicted behaviour at Time 2 (one month later) over and above the effect of behavioural intentions. However, they did not examine the effect of including Time 1 behaviour in the model. Furthermore, their measures of habit and behaviour seem to be problematic in at least two ways. First, the measures may be spuriously related in that not only did they share the same denominator (the frequency of car travel) but also the numerators were related (the number of times one wears a seat belt by force of habit must be less than or equal to the number of times one wears a seat belt). Second, the two items that were combined to create the index of behaviour correlated only 0.17.

An earlier attempt to expand the Fishbein-Ajzen model to include prior behaviour was the study by Bentler and Speckart (1979). They found that recent behaviour (frequency of alcohol, marijuana, or hard drug use in the past two weeks) had a substantial independent effect on current intentions and on behaviour assessed two weeks later. The behaviour-behaviour effect was at least as large as the intention-behaviour effect, suggesting that such behaviours are only partly under the control of intentions. Similarly, Huba, Wingard and Bentler (1981) found that adolescents' intentions to use drugs significantly predicted substance use one year later, but that the increase in prediction over what was predicted by previous drug use was minimal.

A number of other studies have shown independent effects of prior behaviour on future behaviour (e.g. Bagozzi, 1981; Bentler and Speckart, 1981; Fredricks and Dossett, 1983; Godin, Valois and Lepage, 1993; Godin, Valois, Shephard and Desharnais, 1987; Valois, Desharnais and Godin, 1988). To this list should be added the studies we describe in more detail below. Despite such evidence, neither Fishbein nor Ajzen has so far responded by expanding the Theory of Reasoned Action/Planned Behaviour to include prior behaviour as an additional explanatory construct. Indeed, Ajzen (1987) has questioned whether past behaviour can properly be regarded as an explanatory variable. Arguing from a trait viewpoint, he states 'it serves no useful purpose to include past behaviour (a measure of a very specific behavioral disposition) in *causal* models of human action. Yet, this is precisely what some theorists have proposed' (p. 41). Also, on the same page, he says: 'when ... the "trait" used to predict a behavior is the tendency to perform that very behavior, its explanatory power is completely lost'. He makes the same point in the latest exposition of the theory (Ajzen, 1991).

Factors influencing the behaviour-behaviour relationship

Before discussing some concrete examples, we consider a number of factors, including both measurement and substantive factors, that may influence the size, direction, and interpretation of the behaviour-behaviour relationship.

1. The interval between the two waves of measurement

This could range from two minutes to two decades, but in most applied research on health and safety a few weeks or a few months would be more typical. Generally speaking, the longer the interval the greater the chances are that change will occur and the lower the correlation between B1 and B2. However, this will depend on other factors, including the time reference of the measures.

2. The time reference of the behavioural measures

B1 may be a measure of recent behaviour. But how recent? Yesterday? In the last month? In the last two years? It may refer to lifetime experience (e.g. 'How many cigarettes have you smoked in your life?') or to the distant past ('Did you do any exercise when you were at school?'). Or it may include rather vague time references like 'usually' or 'these days' (e.g. 'Do you usually have breakfast?').

3. The nature of the behavioural criterion

The behavioural criterion may be dichotomous, polychotomous, ordinal, or quantitative. It may be a measure of relative frequency ('On what percentage of your journeys do you wear a seat belt?'), absolute frequency ('How many times have you had an accident while riding your motorbike?'), or simply a binary measure of whether the subject has performed some action ('Did you go for a smear test?'). It is well known (or should be) that the maximum correlation and percentage of variance explained is limited by the range and distribution of the variables; in the extreme case of two dichotomous measures with very discrepant proportions, it is not possible to obtain a large positive correlation or (equivalently) to account for a large percentage of the variance (Cohen and Cohen, 1975).

The measures may vary in other ways. The criterion may be highly specific, including references to target, time, and context ('In the last five years, have you tried to give up smoking cigarettes at work?') or less specific, for example dropping the references to the time and target ('Have you tried to give up smoking at work?'). It may be a single item or an aggregated measure (e.g. an index of healthy eating based on several component measures, or a factor score). It may be a behavioural outcome (e.g. weight loss) rather than a behaviour (e.g. cutting out cakes and biscuits). It may be a self-report measure or, less frequently in this field, one based on direct observation of the behaviour or a biochemical marker.

4. The similarity of the behavioural measures

B1 and B2 may be the same measure or two quite different measures differing in any or all of the features mentioned. Their time references may be different and in some cases may overlap. They may be from different domains; for example, uptake of cervical screening may be used to predict uptake of breast screening.

As Ajzen (1991) points out, measures of past and later behaviour are likely to be more similar to each other than they are to measures of attitudes and intentions. (Likewise, measures of attitudes and intentions are likely to be more similar to each other than they are to measures of behaviour.) Thus, the measures of past and later behaviour may have common error variance (method variance) not shared by the measures of attitudes and intentions. This would show up in a path analysis as a residual effect of past behaviour on future behaviour when attitudes and intentions at Time 1 are controlled for. Shared variance due to similarity of measures or other sources can be represented in structural equation models as correlated errors, and with suitable data it is possible to adjust the estimates of the effects of past behaviour, attitudes, and intentions for the presence of such correlated errors. Method effects can be studied more systematically by crossing methods with constructs using the multitrait-multimethod or MTMM approach (Widaman, 1985). So, for example, one could use both interview and self-completion questionnaires to assess intention and behaviour on two occasions. This approach is rarely used in the area of attitude-behaviour relations.

5. The behavioural domain, sample characteristics, and other substantive factors

All of the previous points refer to measurement and design factors. Equally important, however, are substantive factors. Quite simply, more change will occur in some behaviours, samples, times, and circumstances than in others. For example, in the population of adult smokers who also drink, the stability of cigarette consumption may differ from the stability of alcohol consumption. Substantive and measurement factors may be confounded, making it difficult to compare and interpret findings from different behavioural domains. If seat belt use appears more stable than exercising, this may reflect the use of different measures rather than necessarily indicating that these behaviours have different characteristics.

How to maximize the behaviour-behaviour correlation

With reference to the factors outlined above, it is possible to draw up a list of recommendations for maximizing the correlation between B1 and B2: (1) use quantitative measures with many possible values and similar distributions; (2) use identical measures; (3) use a short interval between B1 and B2; (4) use multiple indicators and aggregate to increase reliability (e.g. by latent variable modelling); (5) select the behaviour, the sample, and the conditions such that high stability is expected; (6) make sure that the range of the measures is not restricted; and (7) don't control for any other variables that are correlated positively with B1.

Although the above discussion is meant to be instructive, in practice it is unlikely that a study would have the aim of maximizing the behaviour-behaviour correlation. We would probably be more interested in explaining the behaviour and/or in predicting it from a small number of variables. If these are our aims, the last recommendation in particular should not be taken literally; the other variables referred to will include those that we believe to be important determinants and/or predictors of B2 (e.g. intention, perceived behavioural control), and we will certainly want to include these in the analysis.

The interpretation of a residual effect of B1 on B2 will depend very much on which other variables have been included and which have been omitted from the analysis. If an important variable has been omitted (from the analysis or from the study) and this variable is correlated with B1, then the B1-B2 path will reflect the effect of the omitted variable as well as the true effect of B1 on B2. Ajzen (1991) has suggested that the omission of a measure of perceived behavioural control may account for the effects of past behaviour observed by Bentler and Speckart (1979). However, Godin, Valois and Lepage (1993) have recently reported two applications of the Theory of Planned Behaviour to exercising which showed large effects of past behaviour even when perceived behavioural control was included in the model. It is, of course, always possible after the fact to explain away an effect in terms of omitted variables. Thus, a residual effect of past behaviour can always be explained by invoking an omitted attitudinal variable. Whether this is reasonable depends on whether it can be justified theoretically.

Examples of behaviour-behaviour relationships

Example 1: Taking up smoking

In a prospective study of over 4,000 children, 52 per cent of those who had tried smoking once by age twelve or thirteen had smoked again within two years compared with 36 per cent of those who had not tried smoking at Time 1 (Goddard, 1990; Sutton, 1992). Prior experimentation also emerged as the strongest predictor of smoking uptake in an earlier prospective study even with a measure of intention to smoke in the model (McNeill, Jarvis, Stapleton, Russell, Eiser, Gammage and Gray, 1989).

There are two possible interpretations of this behaviour-behaviour relationship, neither of which is appropriately described by the word habit. The first interpretation says that trying a cigarette has certain consequences (e.g. changes in self-image, changes in beliefs about the effects of smoking, physiological and pharmacological effects) which increase the likelihood of trying a second cigarette. The second interpretation says that if you are predisposed (because of background, personality, attitudes, etc) to try a cigarette, you may be similarly predisposed to smoke again. It is important to be clear that these two explanations are quite different. According to the first explanation, trying the second cigarette is a causal effect of trying the first cigarette, an influence that is mediated via the consequences of the initial act. According to the second explanation, the relationship between B1 and B2 is entirely due to the causal effects of common factors on both. The two kinds of explanation can be applied equally well to experimentation with other substances (e.g. chocolate) and with other activities (e.g. skiing).

Example 2: Giving up smoking

A second example of a behaviour-behaviour relationship for which habit does not appear to provide an appropriate explanation also comes from the smoking field. In a study of 966 cigarette smokers derived from a general population sample, the likelihood of attempting to stop smoking in a six month follow-up period was positively related to the number of previous attempts to quit, even when attitudinal factors were controlled (Sutton, Marsh and Matheson, 1987). Those who had tried more frequently in the past were more likely to try again. Although a large part of the effect was apparently mediated by intentions, there was also a significant direct effect. The first component could be explained as a self-attribution effect (Bem, 1972). Judgements about the likelihood of a future action may be made partly on the basis of past behaviour: 'I've tried to stop smoking before, so it's quite likely I'll try again'. However, it clearly does not make sense to talk about a smoker habitually trying to quit, unless we mean simply that they have done it repeatedly.

Example 3: Breast screening attendance

A recent study of breast screening attendance (Sutton, Bickler, Sancho-Aldridge and Saidi, 1994) provides an interesting example of a negative behaviour-behaviour relationship. The results showed that in a sample of 1,301 women aged 50-64 who were invited for breast screening in the national programme, those who had been before for a breast screen were *less* likely to take up the offer. Further analysis showed that it was those women who had been recently (within the previous twelve months) who were less likely to accept the invitation. The behaviour-behaviour relationship persisted even when intention, perceived importance of breast screening, and other significant predictors were controlled. More generally, one would expect to find negative behaviour-behaviour relationships when the behaviour in question is cyclical or periodic (i.e. a behaviour that is, or should be, repeated at regular intervals), possibly prompted by receiving a postal invitation or other reminder, and when B1 is a measure of recent behaviour. So, for example, a person who has just had her car serviced is unlikely to have it done again in the immediate future. Other factors that may operate to produce negative behaviour-behaviour relationships include satiation and recovery (e.g. getting drunk on Saturday night may reduce one's chances of getting drunk on Sunday night), including economic recovery (you may not be able to afford to go out drinking again), and boredom/curiosity (those who have not tried something before may be more likely to try it, given the opportunity, than those who have already experienced it). In general, aversive experiences are likely to produce negative behaviour-behaviour relationships ('once bitten, twice shy').

Example 4: Seat belt use

In a prospective study of seat belt use conducted in the United Kingdom before legislation was introduced, 456 employees of an agrochemical company in Cambridge completed a short questionnaire and those who wished to participate in a 'health information programme' were then randomly assigned to watching a film about seat belts or a control film (Sutton and Hallett, 1989). Reported seat belt use was measured three months and twelve months after exposure. The results showed strong stability effects. Belt use at three months was related to intentions measured immediately after the film but initial belt use also had a strong independent predictive effect. Similarly, belt use at twelve months was strongly predicted by belt use at three months. We interpreted the results as showing that seat belt use, though influenced in part by beliefs and intentions, has a large habitual component. However, this raises the question of what it means to describe a behaviour as habitual.

Habits

The term habit is perhaps most appropriately used to refer to short sequences of oral-manipulative behaviour that are repeated many times a day and have become autonomous in the sense that they are no longer under the control of the original causal factors. Examples would be thumb sucking, nail biting, playing with worry beads, and (possibly) smoking. In a study of Greek men, it is likely that use of worry beads at Time 1 will strongly predict use of worry beads at Time 2. This relationship can be explained in terms of habit. At least for a proportion of Greek men, worry beads are used so frequently that the behaviour has become autonomous and persists for this reason. This case should be distinguished from the one where the underlying causes persist to maintain the behaviour. The special feature of a habit is that the behaviour continues even when the originating conditions no longer hold. Habits are difficult to change and will often show inconsistency between attitudes and behaviour. For example, we may prefer not to bite our nails but nevertheless carry on doing so because we are unable to stop (the behaviour is not under volitional control). As well as being autonomous, habits are also automatic and subject to intermittent or low levels of awareness.

Some repeated behaviours look like habits but are not autonomous in the way that habits are. If a smoker has a repeated need for the stimulant effect of nicotine and smokes twenty cigarettes a day in response to this need, then it would not be accurate to describe this as habitual smoking, unless we simply wished to point out the high frequency of the behaviour.

Routines

Many behaviours that are referred to as habits in the literature on health behaviours (e.g. seat belt use, taking regular exercise) are more appropriately regarded as routines. A *routine* is a sequence of behaviours that is repeated on a regular basis (e.g. daily, weekly, monthly, yearly). For example, a person's early morning routine may consist of the following actions: get out of bed, take a shower, have a shave, get dressed, have breakfast, drive to work. Each step in the routine can be broken down into a number of separate steps or subroutines. This process can be followed to any level of detail. In the same way, a routine may itself be part of a higher level routine. The advantage of routines is that they save the time and cognitive work that would be involved in repeatedly making the same minor decisions (e.g. 'Would it be better for me to shave first and then have breakfast or to have breakfast first?').

Routinized behaviours are highly predictable over time and may produce large behaviour-behaviour correlations. However, although we may describe someone as 'a creature of habit', meaning that they stick to a regular routine, routine behaviours are not habitual in the sense that nail biting and playing with worry beads are. Although routines are sometimes imposed (e.g. on children by their parents; on army cadets by their officers), in most other cases routines are the result of a deliberate decision to adopt a particular course of action. The routine is sustained by brief self-reminders which serve to reinforce the earlier decision. For example, a man who is concerned about his health may decide to go jogging every morning, or a woman may decide to examine her breasts for lumps once a month. These new routines do not persist of their own accord but have to be maintained by repeated self-reminders. Routines differ in this way from habits that have become autonomous. This may be largely a matter of frequency of repetition; a routine that is repeated many times a day over a period of time may become a habit. More attention should be paid in future research to the frequency and duration of repeated health behaviours.

One test of whether an action is a habit or a routine is whether it is capable of being modified temporarily. If a person who usually eats breakfast at home has to travel to attend an early meeting, she may modify her usual routine just for that day by having breakfast on the train. Another test is whether or not the person sometimes forgets to perform the action at the appropriate time. For example, if a person forgets to switch off the burglar alarm one morning, this would suggest that switching off the alarm is a routine not a habit; presumably, one does not forget habits.

Many routinized behaviours are trivial but others have implications for health and safety. We have mentioned seat belt use, taking regular exercise, and breast self-examination. In addition, many of the behaviours involved in shopping for food and in food preparation and cooking are routinized to eliminate the need for a vast number of minor decisions having to be made anew every day or every week of a person's life.

Non-actions, inertia, procrastination, and postponement

Many behavioural criteria have a 'don't do it' category (e.g. smoke/don't smoke; go jogging/never go jogging). In a general population sample of smokers and non smokers, those who do not smoke at Time 1 will probably also not be smoking at Time 2 (say, three months later), and similarly those who are smoking at Time 1 will probably also be smoking at Time 2. Thus smoking status at Time 1 (B1) will strongly predict smoking status at Time 2 (B2). Continuing not to smoke can hardly be described as a habit or a routine; only positive actions can be described in this way. The term *inertia* is perhaps more appropriate here. If we have never done a particular action, we will tend to carry on not doing it unless there is some cue or invitation or opportunity or reason for trying it. This is particularly the case for uncommon behaviours such as hang-gliding. If we wanted to be sure of demonstrating perfect behavioural stability, we would choose an extremely uncommon behaviour (e.g. 'How many times have you climbed Everest in the last three months?') and measure it on two occasions on a suitable sample (e.g. octogenarians). (Note that the correlation between B1 and B2 would be zero in this case.)

The term inertia can also be applied to positive behaviours. In decision making terms, the alternatives available to the individual always include carrying on as before (the no change option). In making a decision about future action, the course of action being pursued currently may have added weight ('inertia weight'). If there is little to choose between the alternatives in terms of their expected outcomes (they are all equally desirable or undesirable), the current course of action may nevertheless be preferred. The individual may in effect be operating an additional, conservative decision rule, namely 'If in doubt, continue as before'.

Many health related decisions permit the possibility of procrastination and postponement. In the case of *procrastination*, the person makes a decision now to do something in the future (e.g. 'I will stop smoking on my fortieth birthday'). This may be further weakened by making the implementation of the decision conditional on some event (e.g. 'I will stop smoking on my fortieth birthday if I find I can no longer run up three flights of stairs'). In the case of *postponement*, on the other hand, the person defers making the decision until some future date (e.g. 'I don't have to decide now about giving up smoking; I can always think about it next year'). Here the person makes a meta-decision about the timing of the decision without the decision itself being made. The effects of inertia, procrastination, and postponement are the same: to increase the stability of behaviour and dampen the forces for change.

Conclusion

This chapter started with the observation that past behaviour is frequently the best predictor of future behaviour. If we are simply interested in prediction, then we should always employ a suitable measure of past behaviour. Since there is ample evidence that behavioural intentions (or behavioural expectations; see Warshaw and Davis, 1985) also frequently give accurate predictions of future behaviour, then to the extent that they contain independent information, using a measure of past behaviour in combination with a measure of behavioural intentions/expectations is likely to yield a useful level of prediction in most situations. Thus to predict people's behaviour from self-report measures, simply ask them (a) whether/how many times they have done it before and (b) whether they intend or expect to do it in the future. In order to maximize the accuracy of prediction, follow the recommendations made in earlier sections (see also Ajzen and Fishbein, 1980). In addition, prediction of self-report measures should be improved to the extent that subjects are made familiar with the measure of the criterion behaviour (e.g. 'This is the question we will be asking you in three months' time to assess your biscuit consumption. Please indicate what you think your answer will be at that time.').

However, we are usually interested not simply in predicting behaviour but also in explaining it. This involves developing and testing causal models such as the Theory of Planned Behaviour. Research on health and safety behaviours has shown that past behaviour often bypasses intentions and has a residual effect on future behaviour. Similar examples can be found in research in other behavioural domains. In the course of this chapter, we have considered a number of possible interpretations of such findings. To summarize them, an independent effect of past behaviour on future behaviour could reflect: (1) shared method variance in the measures of behaviour; (2) inadequate reliability of the intention measure; (3) changes in intention that occur after (possibly as a result of) initial measurement; (4) failure to translate intention into action owing to lack of volitional control over the behaviour (e.g. because the behaviour is habitual); and (5) omitted attitudinal or other variables correlated with the measure of prior behaviour. Note that none of these interpretations carries the implication that past behaviour directly causes future behaviour.

The above discussion suggests a number of avenues for future research and theory development. The distinction between habits and routines should be developed further. Longitudinal studies that track the adoption, maintenance, and discontinuation of repeated health behaviours, and the accompanying changes in attitudes and intentions, would be particularly valuable. The conditions under which independent effects of past behaviour are observed need to be specified. Methodological studies looking at method effects and other measurement issues in the context of the kinds of self-report measures used to operationalize the Theory of Planned Behaviour would also be worthwhile. Finally, we recommend that researchers who use social psychological models to study health and safety behaviours should 'routinely' include measures of past behaviour, and wherever possible should use multiple indicators of intentions to maximize reliability.

Acknowledgement

I am grateful to the Imperial Cancer Research Fund for continued financial support.

References

Ajzen, I. (1987), 'Attitudes, traits, and actions: dispositional prediction of behavior in personality and social psychology', in Berkowitz, L. (ed.), *Advances in Experimental Social Psychology*, Vol. 20, Academic Press, San Diego.

Ajzen, I. (1988), *Attitudes, Personality, and Behavior*, Open University Press, Milton Keynes.

Ajzen, I. (1991), 'The Theory of Planned Behavior', *Organizational Behavior and Human Decision Processes*, 50, pp. 179-211.

Ajzen, I. and Fishbein, M. (1980), *Understanding Attitudes and Predicting Social Behavior*, Prentice-Hall, Englewood Cliffs, NJ.

Bagozzi, R.P. (1981), 'Attitudes, intentions, and behavior: a test of some key hypotheses', *Journal of Personality and Social Psychology*, 41, pp. 607-627.

Bem, D.J. (1972), 'Self-perception theory', in Berkowitz, L. (ed.), *Advances in Experimental Social Psychology*, Vol. 6, Academic Press, New York.

Bentler, P.M. and Speckart, G. (1979), 'Models of attitude-behavior relations', *Psychological Review*, 86, pp. 452-464.

Bentler, P.M. and Speckart, G. (1981), 'Attitudes "cause" behaviors: a structural equation analysis', *Journal of Personality and Social Psychology*, 40, pp. 226-238.

Campbell, D.T. (1963), 'Social attitudes and other acquired behavioral dispositions', in Koch, S. (ed.), *Psychology: A Study of a Science*, Vol. 6, McGraw-Hill, New York.

Cohen, J. and Cohen, P. (1975), *Applied Multiple Regression/Correlation Analysis for the Behavioral Sciences*, John Wiley and Sons, Hillsdale, NJ.

Fredricks, A.J. and Dossett, D.L. (1983), 'Attitude-behavior relations: a comparison of the Fishbein-Ajzen and the Bentler-Speckart models', *Journal of Personality and Social Psychology*, 45, pp. 501-512.

Goddard, E. (1990), *Why Children Start Smoking*, HMSO, London.

Godin, G., Valois, P. and Lepage, L. (1993), 'The pattern of influence of perceived behavioral control upon exercising behavior: an application of Ajzen's Theory of Planned Behavior', *Journal of Behavioral Medicine*, 16, pp. 81-102.

Godin, G., Valois, P., Shephard, R.J. and Desharnais, R. (1987), 'Prediction of leisure-time exercise behavior: a path analysis (LISREL V) model', *Journal of Behavioral Medicine*, 10, pp. 145-158.

Huba, G.J., Wingard, J.A. and Bentler, P.M. (1981), 'Intentions to use drugs among adolescents: a longitudinal analysis', *International Journal of the Addictions*, 16, pp. 331-339.

Hull, C.L. (1943), *Principles of Behaviour: An Introduction to Behaviour Theory*, Appleton-Century Crofts, New York.

McNeill, A.D., Jarvis, M.J., Stapleton, J.A., Russell, M.A.H., Eiser, J.R., Gammage, P. and Gray, E.M. (1989), 'Prospective study of factors predicting uptake of smoking in adolescents', *Journal of Epidemiology and Community Health*, 43, pp. 72-78.

Ronis, D.L., Yates, J.F., and Kirscht. J.P. (1989), 'Attitudes, decisions, and habits as determinants of repeated behavior', in Pratkanis, A.R., Breckler, S.J. and Greenwald, A.G. (eds), *Attitude Structure and Function*, Erlbaum, Hillsdale, NJ, pp. 213-239.

Sutton, S.R. (1992), 'Is taking up smoking a reasoned action?', *British Journal of Addiction*, 87, pp. 21-24.

Sutton, S.R., Bickler, G., Sancho-Aldridge, J. and Saidi, G. (1994), 'Prospective study of predictors of attendance for breast screening in an inner-city area', *Journal of Epidemiology and Community Health*, in press.

Sutton, S.R. and Hallett, R. (1989), 'Understanding seat-belt intentions and behavior: a decision-making approach', *Journal of Applied Social Psychology*, 19, pp. 1310-1325.

Sutton, S.R., Marsh, A. and Matheson, J. (1987), 'Explaining smokers' decisions to stop: test of an expectancy-value approach', *Social Behaviour*, 2, pp. 35-49.

Triandis, H.C. (1977), *Interpersonal Behavior*, Brooks/Cole, Monterey, CA.

Valois, P., Desharnais, R. and Godin, G. (1988), 'A comparison of the Fishbein and Ajzen and the Triandis attitudinal models for the prediction of exercise intention and behavior', *Journal of Behavioral Medicine*, 11, pp. 459-472.

Warshaw, P.R. and Davis, F.D. (1985), 'Disentangling behavioral intention and behavioral expectation', *Journal of Experimental Social Psychology*, 21, pp. 213-228.

Widaman, K.F. (1985), 'Hierarchically nested covariance structure models for multitrait-multimethod data', *Applied Psychological Measurement*, 9, pp. 1-26.

Wittenbraker, J., Gibbs, B.L. and Kahle, L.R. (1983), 'Seat belt attitudes, habits, and behaviors: an adaptive amendment to the Fishbein model', *Journal of Applied Social Psychology*, 13, pp. 406-421.

5 Relations among variables influencing drivers' intentions to drive after drinking

Lars Åberg

Introduction

Road accidents constitute a serious health problem all over the world (Evans, 1991). Results from road accident investigations show that human errors dominate among causes of car crashes (Rumar, 1985). However, each accident is the result of a unique chain of events which are both unexpected and rare, and to state the causes of accidents is difficult. Many accidents are the result of occasional deviations from drivers' normal activities, and one way to acquire knowledge about the processes that increase the risk of accidents would therefore be to study the factors that influence drivers' behaviour in normal, everyday traffic situations.

Many efforts have been made to analyse driver behaviour by psychological models (see Michon, 1985, for a review), but there is great variation among the models concerning the theoretical origins of behaviour. One widely used approach has been the Theory of Reasoned Action (Ajzen and Fishbein, 1980) — which focuses on motivational aspects of volitional behaviour — and it is this that provides the framework for the present chapter. The model has already been used as a conceptual framework in several studies of accident-related driver behaviours, including drink-driving, use of safety belts and other safety devices, and speed adjustment (e.g. Wittenbraker, Gibbs and Kahle, 1982; Vogel and Rothengatter, 1984; Rutter, Quine and Chesham, 1990; Åberg, 1993).

The Theory of Reasoned Action and causal analysis

The Theory of Reasoned Action (TRA) is generally represented as a path diagram, and it therefore invites the use of advanced statistical methods for the analysis of data. Causal modelling (see Pedhazur, 1982) is an elaborated form of path analysis, and one frequently applied method for causal modelling is LISREL analysis (Jöreskog and Sörbom, 1989). In LISREL a causal model of latent (unobserved) variables is postulated, and the latent structure is connected to observed variables via a measurement model. A comparison is then made between predictions from the model and empirical data, and a test of significance is used to reach a decision concerning the fit between the theoretical model and the observed data.

The procedure of causal analysis normally involves several steps. In an initial analysis the model is tested against a set of empirical data. If the fit is not good the original causal model is revised until a better fit is obtained, but if it is not possible to reach an acceptable fit, the original model has to be rejected. When a revised model is accepted it must be cross-validated on a new sample of subjects to avoid capitalization on chance. The purpose of the present chapter is to present the results of a LISREL analysis performed on data from a questionnaire study of drink-driving intentions and behaviour.

Investigation of drivers' opinions and experiences of drink-driving

Drink-driving is generally considered one of the most important causes of traffic accidents, and the risk of accidents increases steeply with increasing levels of alcohol in the blood (e.g. Evans, 1991). To improve traffic safety it is important to find measures to prevent drink-driving, measures that should rely on knowledge about factors influencing people's decisions to drive after consuming alcohol. Drink-driving is the focus of the present study.

In 1987 a questionnaire designed to investigate drink-driving and based on the TRA was distributed to a random sample of 4,100 Swedish drivers (see Åberg, 1993, for further details). It included questions about TRA variables such as previous and intended drink-driving, attitudes, and social norms, and also evaluations related to drink-driving and expectations about sanctions and about the consequences of accidents. The behaviour of interest was defined as drink-driving violations during a three year period. There were also questions concerning sex, age, drinking habits, driving habits, work situation, and factors describing circumstances when decisions to drive after drinking were made. Sixty per cent of the questionnaires were returned, yielding a sample of 2,490 subjects. Among the drivers a subgroup of 1,085 non-teetotal male drivers between 18 and 55 years of age were selected and their data subjected to a LISREL analysis.

A hierarchical latent variable structure in accordance with the standard TRA was used as the starting point for the analyses (see Figure 5.1). According to criteria given in the statistical procedure the initial model

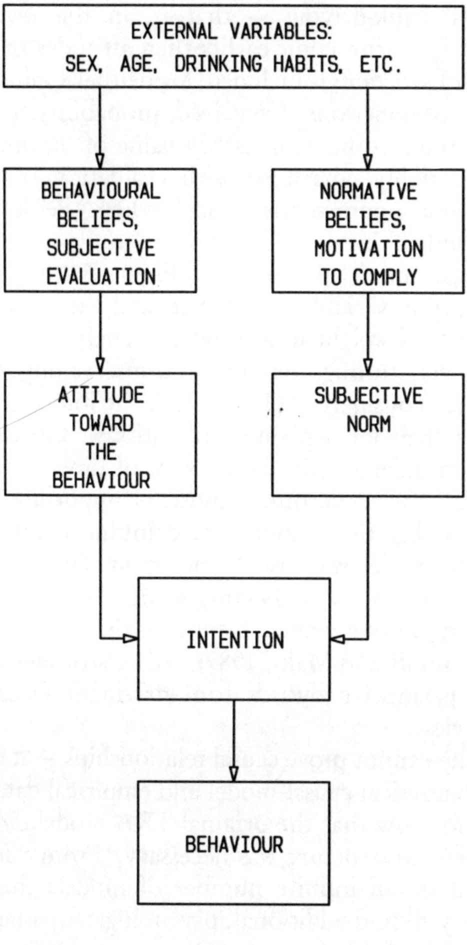

Figure 5.1 The TRA model. After Ajzen (1980)

was modified to obtain a structure that fitted the empirical data and at the same time explained as much of the behavioural variance as possible (for details see Åberg, 1993). The cross-validated, revised model for the structure of latent variables is presented in Figure 5.2.

The revised latent structure is different from the TRA model. It includes a dependent variable that is a combination of intentions and previous behaviour. Also, social norms precede personal evaluations as well as attitudes towards drink-driving — that is, in the revised model it is suggested that social norms come earlier than attitudes in the causal chain. Only evaluation of *sanctions* is included, for neither evaluation of accidents nor expectation of sanctions (perceived probability of detection) and accidents contributed to the explanatory value of the model. Evaluation of accidents was highly correlated with evaluation of punishment and could therefore not improve the model when the latter variable had already been included.

In the final causal model presented in Figure 5.2, an arrow indicates a direct effect from one variable to another, and the strength of the effect is equivalent to a beta weight in a regression analysis. Indirect effects are represented by effects through one or more intervening variables. If only direct effects are considered (Table 5.1), attitudes emerge as more important than norms for explaining intentions. On the other hand, if total effects are considered, that is the sum of direct and indirect effects (Table 5.2), social norms become almost as important as attitudes. It should be noticed that the influence of drinking habits in the model is very strong. The model was also found to fit data obtained in parallel questionnaire investigations in Denmark and Norway, although drink-driving is much more frequent in Denmark than in Sweden or Norway (Åberg, Glad, Bernhoft and Mäki, 1989). Also, attitudes and social norms were much more permissive towards drink-driving in Denmark than in the other two countries.

Causal modelling cannot prove causal relationships — it can only indicate a fit between a theoretical causal model and empirical data. In the present case it was used to show that the original TRA model did not fit the data well and that a revised structure was necessary. From a *statistical* point of view there might be an infinite number of models that fit data. It is therefore necessary to find additional, psychologically plausible, reasons to justify any revised model before it can be accepted as an explanation. In the remaining part of this chapter, possible explanations for the differences between the TRA model and the revised model will be discussed.

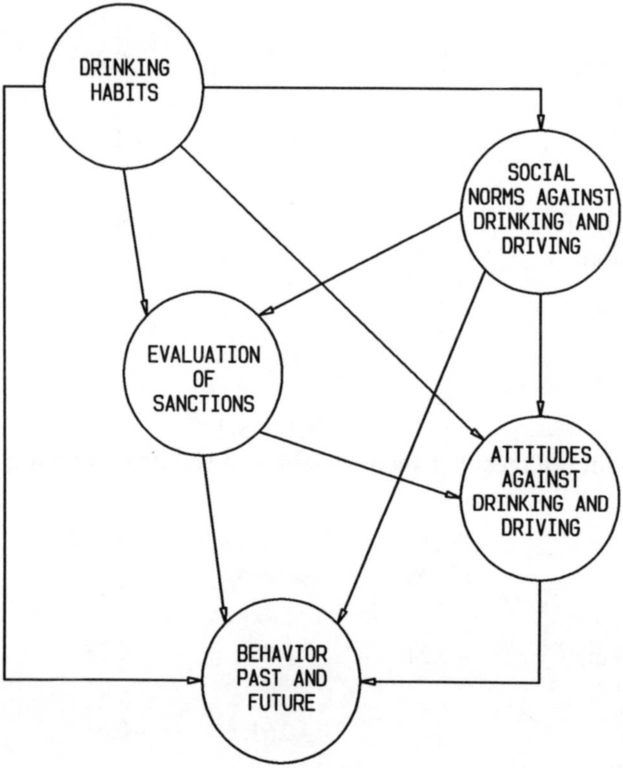

Figure 5.2 The drink-driving model of latent variables. The arrows indicate direct influences among variables

Table 5.1
Path coefficients indicating direct effects between variables in the drink-driving model

	Social Norm	Evaluation Sanction	Attitude	Behaviour-Intention
Drinking Habits	-0.21	0.17	0.22	0.29
Social Norm	—	-0.51	-0.39	-0.09
Evaluation Sanction	—	—	0.27	0.14
Attitude	—	—	—	0.52

Table 5.2
Total effects between variables in the drink-driving model

	Social Norm	Evaluation Sanction	Attitude	Behaviour-Intention
Drinking Habits	-0.21	0.28	0.38	0.54
Social Norm	—	-0.51	-0.53	-0.44
Evaluation Sanction	—	—	0.27	0.28
Attitude	—	—	—	0.52

Social norms and attitudes in the Theory of Reasoned Action

One reason for the deviation of the present solution from the original TRA model might be that the latter was not appropriately designed for causal analysis. In the TRA there is no path between attitudes and social norms, indicating that there is little or no correlation. However, in studies reported by Ajzen and Fishbein (1980) and Ajzen (1985) the results point to a substantial relationship between the two variables, something that would justify a causal path in one direction or the other. According to Rothengatter (1991), the Theory of Reasoned Action is a static model, adequate for describing motives underlying behaviour but not designed to predict behavioural change. This would explain the lack of interest in postulating a link between attitudes and social norms. In a model prepared for causal analysis of influences from external variables, via beliefs, attitudes, and social norms to intention and behaviour, it is necessary to include a path between attitude and social norms until the variables are proved to be unrelated. In the present causal analysis it proved essential to include such a path. From a psychological point of view the most likely causal direction was considered to be social norm, via evaluation of punishment, to attitude. In the next section, arguments in favour of social norm as a cause of attitudes towards safe behaviour and rule compliance will be presented.

Social norms, safe behaviour and rule compliance

Even for someone who drives faster than the speed limits, who fails to use a safety belt, or who drives after drinking too much, the probability of an accident is very small. For example, the probability that an average Swedish driver will be involved in a fatal accident is estimated to be less than one in 5,000 years, and for an injury accident it is less than one in 200 years. It is therefore unlikely that a driver will have the opportunity to form expectations and to learn about the consequences of accidents from his or her own experiences. Much the same applies to law-breaking. For example, even if a Swedish driver constantly drives 15 km/h over the speed limit he is unlikely to be detected more than once every three years. Similarly, he can drive for five years before he is likely to be stopped for a breath test. Thus, what most drivers will learn by experience is that there are many things they can do in traffic without experiencing an accident or punishment. Nevertheless, most drivers wear seat belts, many do not violate speed limits and very few (at least in Sweden) drive after consuming alcohol. However, if risk evaluations are important for decisions in traffic and if drivers cannot be expected to learn from experience about the likelihood and consequences of accidents and sanctions, how do they acquire their values and expectations?

One possible answer is that people learn from others, and several authors have also claimed that social norms affect judgements of risk (e.g. Simpson, 1990; Evans, 1991). In investigations in Uppsala drivers were asked to rate various consequences of drink-driving and speeding (Åberg, 1990; Haglund and Åberg, 1994). Being suspected of drink-driving but not being punished was rated as more negative than being fined for speeding. Losing one's driving licence for drink-driving or speeding was rated just as negatively as being involved in an injury accident or going to jail for drink-driving. Drivers rated injuring other people as significantly more negative than injuring themselves. Thus it is not easy to see a direct relationship between the evaluation of consequences and the direct personal effects of those consequences.

A further point of interest comes from recent Swedish legislation. A change in the blood alcohol limit from 0.05 per cent to 0.02 per cent in 1990 was met with strong approval in the public debate although the law will probably not have an effect on traffic safety (Evans 1991). At the same time, however, public opinion favoured raising speed limits, which is likely to increase the number of injuries in traffic (Nilsson, 1991). Actual risks in traffic thus appear not to be directly related to drivers' evaluations of dangerous behaviours. A possible explanation is that social or moral norms are more important than drivers' own experiences of risk. I should like to propose that this may offer indirect support for a structural model in which social norms precede evaluations of sanctions and accidents.

Perceived probability of detection

In the TRA model the sum of the products of personal beliefs and evaluations of behavioural consequences is assumed to determine attitude. In the present model of drink-driving, evaluation of sanctions was found to be a latent variable. It was also assumed that expectations about being detected would improve the model because studies of the effects of police enforcement (e.g. Nilsson and Åberg, 1986) have shown that the probability of detection covaries significantly with behaviour, both for speeding and for drink-driving. However, the perceived probability of detection was not found to improve the present model, either in interaction with evaluations or as a single variable. This is in agreement with the result of another study of drink-driving in Sweden (Norström, 1983), in which moral issues and alcohol consumption were the main determinants of drink-driving, while the probability of detection had no effect.

The fact that perceived probability of detection did not improve the present model may be related to the way in which the target behaviour was defined. It is well known that there is considerable variation in the subjective probability of detection in relation to the time of day or week and the particular environment (Åberg, Engdahl and Nilsson, 1986), for drivers have a good idea when and where the police are likely to be patrolling. Drink-driving is very infrequent and therefore, in the questionnaire study, subjects were asked about their drink-driving experiences during a period of three years. If behaviour is aggregated over a long period, including variations over times and places, the predictive power of the perceived probability of detection will decrease, and the model will not be improved.

From a more recent investigation of drink-driving (Åberg, 1992), evidence has emerged that *beliefs* might be important for decisions to drink and drive. On 1 July 1990, in Sweden, the blood alcohol concentration limit was changed from 0.05 per cent to 0.02 per cent, as we have seen. To evaluate the change, the questionnaire investigation from 1987 was repeated in 1991 on a new sample of 2,100 drivers (Åberg, 1992). Again answers were obtained from 60 per cent. Preliminary results showed that very little had changed since the introduction of the new limit, for the drivers reported the same drinking habits and the same drink-driving behaviour as four years earlier. However, they reported more violations of the law than in 1987, and they expected they would violate the law more often after implementation of the lower limit. Although attitudes towards violations were still negative, they were significantly less negative than before the new limit, and there was a significant decrease in the perceived probabilities of accidents and detection. Thus, the new law can be seen to have influenced a number of variables that were in the model and also some that had been excluded.

Intention and behaviour

The present drink-driving model included past behaviour. The results show a high covariation between past behaviour and intentions. Subjects were asked about the number of drink-driving violations they had committed during the last three years and were asked to rate the probability that they would drink and drive in the next three years. The analysis showed that the answers to the two kinds of questions could be explained by a single latent variable: drivers who reported previous drink-driving also expected to drive when drunk in the future. Even though these drivers were not as negative as other drivers in their attitudes towards drink-driving, they were still negative to some extent. Drinking habits were found to be as important as attitudes for drink-driving (see Table 5.2), probably because of the increased number of situations in which drivers have to decide whether to drive or not. Perhaps the inclusion of another variable, 'perceived behavioural control' suggested by Ajzen (1991) in his Theory of Planned Behaviour, would have been appropriate for tapping this particular issue. According to the Theory of Planned Behaviour, perceived behavioural control provides a link between past and future behaviour, and might well discriminate between drivers who drink and drive and those who do not. It will be interesting to include perceived behavioural control in future studies.

Concluding remarks

The study of drink-driving reported in this chapter has shown that attitudes and social norms, as well as drinking habits, are important for predicting and understanding drink-driving. An attempt to find a causal model that could explain the behaviour was successful, but it was different from the TRA model used as a frame of reference for the study. In the TRA the path between attitudes and social norms is assumed to be close to zero, while in the model presented here subjective norm precedes evaluations and attitudes. The structure has been found to be stable over a number of samples. LISREL analysis alone cannot say anything about the order of variables or direction of influences in a causal structure like the present one, but the order of variables we have suggested is in accordance with other observations concerning driver behaviour, for example perceived risks in traffic. The result is also in agreement with the reasoning of authors who stress the importance of social influences on drivers' decision making (e.g. Evans, 1991; Simpson, 1990; Rothengatter, 1991).

One factor known from other investigations to affect drivers' decision making is the perceived probability of detection. This particular measure did not enter the present model, probably because perceived probabilities even out over time and space and so make no contribution to the explanation of behaviour. According to Ajzen and Fishbein (1980), the perceived probability of detection would be a better predictor for a behaviour clearly specified in time and space, and in those circumstances the TRA model might be more appropriate.

In the present model, past behaviour and intention for future behaviour were explained by a single latent variable. As drink-driving is considered very negative, even among those who do it, 'expected future behaviour' might be a more suitable term to use than intention (Warshaw and Davis, 1985). A driver who in the past has driven after drinking expects that he will do so again, simply because of his drinking habits. Similar arguments have been made elsewhere in this volume, and they are set to have an important influence on future research, not least in road safety.

References

Åberg, L. (1990), 'Bilförares beslutsfattande i anslutning till alkoholförtäring. Enkätstudie', Swedish Transport Research Board, *TFB-meddelande 170*.

Åberg, L. (1992), 'Behaviours and opinions of Swedish drivers before and after the 0.02 per cent legal BAC limit of 1990', paper presented at the ICADTS-t'92 Conference, Cologne, Germany, 1992.

Åberg, L. (1993), 'Drinking and driving: intentions, attitudes and social norms of Swedish male drivers', *Accident Analysis and Prevention*, 25, pp. 289-296.

Åberg, L., Glad, A., Bernhoft, I.M. and Mäki, M. (1990), 'Social norms, attitudes and intentions concerning drinking and driving. A cross-national comparison', in Perrine, M.W.B. (ed.), *Proceedings of the 11th International Conference on Alcohol, Drugs and Traffic Safety*, National Safety Council, Chicago.

Ajzen, I. (1985), 'From intentions to actions: a theory of planned behaviour', in Kuhl, J. and Beckman, J. (eds), *Action Control: From Cognition to Behaviour*, Springer, Heidelberg.

Ajzen, I. (1991), 'The Theory of Planned Behavior', *Organizational Behaviour and Human Decision Processes*, 50, pp. 179-211.

Ajzen, I. and Fishbein, M. (1980), *Understanding Attitudes and Predicting Social Behaviour*, Prentice Hall, New Jersey.

Evans, L. (1991), *Traffic Safety and the Driver*, Van Nostrand Reinhold, New York.

Haglund, M. and Åberg, L. (1994), 'Stabilitet och generaliserbarhet i förares beteende: egenskaper i mått på hastighet', Swedish Transport Research Board (in press).

Jöreskog, K.G. and Sörbom, D. (1989), *LISREL 7 — A Guide to the Program and Applications*, Second Edition, SPSS Publications, Chicago.

Michon, J.A. (1985), 'A critical view of driver behaviour models. What do we know, what shall we do?', in Evans, L. and Schwing, R. (eds), *Human Behaviour and Traffic Safety*, Plenum Press, New York.

Nilsson, E. and Åberg, L. (1986), 'Övervakning och Påföljd', *TFD-forskning 1976-1983*, Swedish Transport Research Board, 11, Liber distribution, Stockholm.

Nilsson, G. (1991), *Hastigheter, olycksrisker och personskadekonsekvenser i olika vägmiljöer*, Swedish Road and Traffic Research Institute, VTI-meddelande 690.

Norström, T. (1983), 'Law enforcement and alcohol consumption policy as countermeasures against drunken driving: possibilities and limitations', *Accident Analysis and Prevention*, 15, pp. 513-521.

Pedhazur, E.J. (1982), *Multiple Regression in Behavioral Research. Explanation and Prediction*, Second edition, Holt, Reinhart and Winston, New York.

Rothengatter, J.A. (1991), 'Normative behaviour is unattractive if it is abnormal: relationships between norms, attitudes and traffic law', in Koornstra, M.J., and Christensen, J. (eds), *Proceedings of the International Road Safety Symposium in Copenhagen, Denmark, September 19-21, 1990*, SWOV Institute for Road Safety Research, Leidschendam, The Netherlands.

Rumar, K. (1985), 'The role of perceptual and cognitive filters in observed behavior', in Evans, L. and Schwing, R.C. (eds), *Human Behavior and Traffic Safety*, Plenum Press, New York, pp. 151-165.

Rutter, D., Quine, L. and Chesham, D.J. (1990), 'Do motorcyclists' beliefs predict accident liability?', in Benjamin, T. (ed.), *Driving Behaviour in a Social Context*, Paradigme, Caen.

Simpson, H.M. (1990), 'Importing and exporting countermeasures: cultural determinants of success', in Perrine, B.M.W. (ed.), *Alcohol, Drugs and Traffic Safety. Proceedings of the 11th International Conference on Alcohol, Drugs and Traffic Safety*, National Safety Council, Chicago.

Vogel, R. and Rothengatter, J.A. (1984), *Motieven van snelheidsgedrag op autosnelwegen; een attitude onderzog*, Traffic Research Centre, University of Groningen, Haren.

Warshaw, P.R. and Davis, F.D. (1985), 'Disentangling behavioral intention and behavioral expectation', *Journal of Experimental Social Psychology*, 21, pp. 213-228.

Wittenbraker, J., Gibbs, B.L. and Kahle, L.R. (1983), 'Seat belt attitudes, habits, and behaviors: an adaptive amendment to the Fishbein model', *Journal of Applied Psychology*, 13, pp. 406-421.

6 Predicting helmet use among schoolboy cyclists: An application of the Health Belief Model

Laurence Arnold and Lyn Quine

Introduction

The purpose of this chapter is to report a prospective study in which health beliefs were used to predict the use of protective helmets among young cyclists. Many cyclists receive head injuries on British roads each year, especially young cyclists, and many of the injuries are serious or even fatal. In 1991 a total of 24,803 cyclists were injured in the United Kingdom, 2,722 aged between 8 and 11 and 7,569 between 12 and 19; 466 of the 8-11 year olds and 1,191 of the 12-19 year olds were *seriously* injured or killed. Sixty-nine young people between the ages of 8 and 19 died. Apart from injuries from other causes, only cancer claimed more lives in the 8-15 age group. Moreover, there is worrying evidence that casualty rates for pedal cyclists are under-reported. A study for the Department of Transport by Mills (1989) found that 68 per cent of a sample of pedal cycle casualties at a hospital were injured in accidents that had not been reported to the police. Though all *fatal* accidents were reported, 61 per cent of accidents resulting in serious injury and 74 per cent of those resulting in slight injury were not (Mills, 1989).

Overall risks of injury to children in road traffic accidents rise sharply with age. A review by Jones (1989) shows that the casualty rate per 100,000 population doubles when children first enter school, rises again for children of middle school age, and is yet higher for senior age groups. A similar pattern is seen for each severity of injury. Rates of child pedal cyclists killed or seriously injured are close to zero for the very young, but rise markedly when children begin school, and then roughly double with each succeeding age band — to middle school, and on to senior school. Children aged twelve and above may of course travel further to school, with consequently greater exposure to injury than younger children, and that may in part account for the figures. Accurate exposure figures, however, are not available, but the accident rate for boys is six times that for girls, possibly reflecting boys' greater enthusiasm for cycling. Coupled with the observed pattern of accident rates increasing with age, this suggests that boy cyclists in the twelve and over age group are a particularly high risk category (Jones, 1989).

Many child and adolescent cycling accidents are 'school related' — that is, they occur on weekdays on journeys to or from school. For example, in 1989, a fifth of all casualties to pedal cyclists aged ten to fourteen occurred on journeys to school. Child pedal cyclist casualties over the age of ten have a morning peak between 8 and 9 am and an afternoon and early evening peak from 3 pm to 8 pm depending upon age (Taylor, 1989). Pedal cycle casualties to children aged ten to fourteen occur overwhelmingly on built up roads (92 per cent), in daylight (88 per cent), and at junctions (69 per cent).

There is ample evidence that accidents to cyclists can and often do result in serious head injuries. A study of cycling accidents in Australia by Wood and Milne (1986) found that head injuries constituted 33 per cent of reported injuries and accounted for 80 per cent of fatalities. McDermot and Klug (1982) compared the pattern of injuries for motor cyclists (who wore helmets) and pedal cyclists (who did not). The incidences of concussion, fractured base and vault of skull, and inter-cranial trauma were significantly higher in pedal cyclists than in motorcyclists. Stutts, Williamson, Whitley and Sheldon (1990) found that all the fatally injured cyclists in their survey suffered a head injury, and that none of them wore a helmet.

The idea that cycle helmets will help prevent or lessen the severity of head injury finds support in a number of studies (Wood and Milne, 1986; Pitt, Thomas, Nixon, Clark, Battistutta and Acton, 1994). In a case control study of children presenting with bicycle related injuries, Thomas, Acton, Nixon, Battistutta, Pitt and Clark (1994) found that wearing a helmet reduced the risk of head injury by 63 per cent and the risk of loss of consciousness by 86 per cent. Dorsch, Woodward and Somers (1987) concluded from their survey that hard helmets were nineteen times better than no helmet at all. Williams (1990, 1991) tested the response of cycle helmets to simulated impacts and also analysed the performance of helmets worn by cyclists involved in accidents. He concluded that both hard shell and expanded polystyrene foam helmets reduce the risk of head injury effectively, by dispersing the force of impact.

Few cyclists wear helmets. Stutts et al. (1990) found that only 7 per cent of their sample over the age of fifteen, and less than 1 per cent of those under fifteen, wore a helmet. Although some schools encourage their use, the decision is left largely to the individual cyclist. From a social psychological perspective this makes the study of the cyclists' behaviour (wearing or not wearing helmets) more interesting since it is likely to arise from cyclists' beliefs rather than regulations or the insistence of others. Parents or schoolteachers who insist on a helmet being worn against the wishes of the cyclist are likely to be disobeyed once out of sight, so that even the influence of 'powerful others' may need to accord with the cyclist's other beliefs if a helmet is to be worn consistently.

Does social psychological theory have anything to contribute to the understanding of road safety behaviour in children? Recently, theoretical models from social psychology have been applied to a number of road user behaviours, taking beliefs and attitudes as a means of predicting preventive health and safety behaviours. The Theory of Reasoned Action (Fishbein and Ajzen, 1975), its recent extension the Theory of Planned Behaviour (Ajzen, 1988), and the Health Belief Model (Rosenstock, 1966) have all been used with success in understanding road user behaviour, for example wearing seatbelts (Wittenbraker, Gibbs and Kahle, 1983; Budd, North and Spencer, 1984; Budd and Spencer, 1986; Grube, Morgan and McGree, 1986; Nelson and Moffitt, 1988; Sutton and Hallett, 1989; Stasson and Fishbein, 1990); using car seats and restraints for children (Gielen, Eriksen, Dulbray and Rist, 1984; Webb, Sanson-Fisher and Bauman, 1988); avoiding drink-riding (Åberg, in this volume); and avoiding motorcycling accidents (Rutter, Quine and Chesham, 1993). The aim of our present study was to try to predict helmet use in a sample of school aged children, using a prospective design in which beliefs and attitudes towards helmet wearing were measured one month before the dependent measure, actual wearing of a helmet. To guide the structuring of our measures and analyses, we used the Health Belief Model. In addition, we hypothesized that an expanded model adding the Multidimensional Health Locus of Control Scale, a measure of past behaviour, and the subject's age would significantly increase the predictive power of the Health Belief Model.

The Health Belief Model

The Health Belief Model (HBM), originally developed by Rosenstock (1966), was chosen to investigate the relationships between health beliefs and behaviour. Rosenstock's version of the model proposes that people will be motivated to undertake preventive health behaviour in response to a perceived threat to their health such as sustaining serious head injury during a road traffic accident. The Health Belief Model is an expectancy-value approach to health-related decisions (Becker, Drachman and Kirscht, 1972a) and has been described as the oldest (Mullen, Hersey and Iverson,

1987), most widely used (Champion and Miller, 1992), and most scrutinized model (Kelly, Zyzanski and Alemagno, 1991) for investigating health-related behaviour. Rosenstock's model (1966, 1974) drew on motivational principles from Lewin's (1935) field theory, and proposed that preventive health behaviour could be explained by two classes of variables: '(1) the psychological state of readiness to take specific action, and (2) the extent to which a particular course of action is believed to be beneficial in reducing the threat' (Rosenstock, 1966, p. 98). Thus, 'health behaviour is a function of a health motive or threat and the individual's beliefs about various courses of action open to him' (Rosenstock, 1966, p. 297). Since readiness to act is a function of a perceived threat to health, the model is a disease avoidance model concerned with health protective behaviour.

Rosenstock (1966) describes both classes of variables as two dimensional, with an individual's state of readiness to act determined by perceptions of personal susceptibility or *vulnerability* to a particular health threat, and by perceptions of the *severity* with which that threat might affect his or her life. Similarly, the extent to which a course of action is believed to be beneficial is the result of beliefs about the *benefits* to be gained by an action (i.e. its efficacy in reducing the threat) weighed against the costs of, or *barriers* to, action. According to Rosenstock (1966), 'the level of readiness (susceptibility and severity) provides the energy or force to act and the perceptions of benefits (less barriers) provides a preferred path of action' (p. 101). Also of importance is some kind of stimulus or cue to action to trigger the decision making process. This cue can be internal in the form of symptoms or bodily states, or external in the form of personal experiences or advice on, and media exposure to, health matters.

A second version of the model was developed by Becker and his colleagues (Becker, Drachman and Kirscht, 1972a, 1972b, 1974; Becker and Maiman, 1975; Becker, Haefner, Kasl, Kirscht, Maiman and Rosenstock, 1977; Becker, Maiman, Kirscht, Haefner and Drachman, 1977) to investigate 'sick-role behaviour' ('the activity undertaken by those who consider themselves ill for the purpose of getting well', (Kasl and Cobb, 1966)), which was said to 'borrow heavily' from the earlier formulation (Becker et al., 1974, p. 206). Many researchers mistakenly believe that Becker and his associates merely amended Rosenstock's (1966) model by introducing new variables, and that the two versions are thus no more than variations on a theme. In fact the models are based upon quite different motivational principles and as a consequence utilize different variables. They also conceptualize the variables they do have in common in different ways. Although Becker, Maiman, Kirscht, Haefner and Drachman's (1977) model is seldom used, a composite model has evolved (see for example King, 1982; Champion, 1984; McCallum, Wiebe and Keith, 1988; Nemcek, 1990) in which variables from Becker et al.'s version are added to Rosenstock's original. This practice ignores the implications of using the additional variables and often obscures their origins. In addition, different researchers operationalize both the basic and composite models in different ways.

Becker et al. (1972a, 1972b, 1974) proposed that *three* classes of variables determined an individual's readiness to act and thus added a third set of variables measuring 'health motivation' to Rosenstock's 'perceived threat' and 'preferred course of action'. The model then underwent a number of further amendments (Becker, 1974; Becker and Maiman, 1975; Becker et al., 1974) and was later applied to preventive health behaviour (Becker and Maiman, 1975; Becker, Haefner, Kasl, Kirscht, Maiman and Rosenstock, 1977; Becker, Maiman, Kirscht, Haefner and Drachman, 1977), until it eventually differed from Rosenstock's (1966) Health Belief Model in a number of important ways. For example, Rosenstock's 'benefits' dimension was expanded to include additional variables such as 'perceived control' and 'faith in doctors', while 'barriers to action' was moved elsewhere in the model. Severity and vulnerability were combined in an expanded 'threat' dimension, which as well as measuring general and specific vulnerability included 'worry about illnesses'. Finally, a host of non-attitudinal variables were introduced in the guise of modifying and enabling factors.

The most important change was the introduction of a specific measure of 'health motivation', described originally as 'different degrees of readiness to undertake a health action, aroused by health cues' (Becker et al., 1972b, p. 853). Although health motivation was initially thought to operate in conjunction with Rosenstock's two sets of determinants, Becker and Maiman (1975) later invoked a reworking of Atkinson and Feather's (1966) theory of 'achievement motivation' and described health motivation as 'providing the "push factor" in compliance' (p. 18). This effectively relegates Rosenstock's (1966) 'readiness to act' to a secondary influence on health related behaviour and introduces the notion that health behaviour is determined not so much by a threat to health as by an individual's *dispositional* 'need to achieve' (Atkinson and Feather, 1966), which exerts a constant influence across different situations irrespective of the salience of a health threat.

Despite these theoretical implications, health motivation is usually referred to simply as an amendment to the original model and is tacked onto Rosenstock's (1966) variables where it is used as another predictor variable. It can be seen though that this practice in fact introduces a non-specific global measure into a threat specific model, thus radically changing the underlying premise that health behaviour is a function of beliefs specific to a health threat. There are practical problems too, since researchers set out to measure health motivation yet use items that in reality concern the general value of health, concern over health, and/or future intention, which would seem to measure influences other than motivation. Furthermore, a number of researchers (Hill et al., 1985; McCallum et al., 1988; Champion, 1987; Nemcek, 1990) have found that health motivation is *not* a significant predictor of preventive health behaviour. Of the thirty-five studies reviewed for our chapter twenty describe health motivation as an essential part of the Health Belief Model, while the remaining fifteen contain no references to it at all.

In addition to these changes, the research of Becker and his colleagues also initiated a move away from the phenomenological orientation inherent in Rosenstock's (1966) conceptualization. Rosenstock (1960, 1966) argued that an individual acts in response to the environment as he or she perceives it. Thus an initial 'modal' survey of individuals' beliefs is essential to ensure that the measured beliefs reflect the subjective perceptions of the sample. Becker and Maiman's (1975) and Becker, Maiman, Kirscht, Haefner and Drachman's (1977) model encouraged the tendency to measure whatever practical and structural influences on health behaviour the researchers themselves deemed salient despite the fact that they may have little significance for the subjects themselves. Melnyk (1988), in her review, notes that the barriers dimension is more often operationalized as systems characteristics (presumed to act as barriers by the researchers), than as the consumer's perceptions of the subjective costs inherent in a health threat (p. 197).

Of far greater significance, Becker's reconceptualization radically altered the nature of perceived barriers to action and appears to have set a precedent. By being placed among the modifying variables, barriers ceased to be a set of subjective psychological beliefs and instead became a collection of objective structural costs. This would seem contrary to theory, since usually such factors as time, transport, accessibility, and expense will not become apparent (and thus be salient) until an individual attempts the behaviour in question. Such factors should not therefore be viewed as belonging to an initial set of predictors and are probably best measured instead at Time 2 (in prospective studies) since they mediate between intention and behaviour. King (1982), for example, accounts for the discrepancy between the behavioural intent of her subjects and their behaviour by proposing that practical barriers intervened between Time 1 and Time 2. Clarke, Hill, Rassaby, White and Hirst (1991) found that practical barriers were perceived as greater obstacles to performing breast self-examination when measured at Time 2 (after subjects had attempted the behaviour) than when measured at Time 1. With regard to preventive behaviours that involve an initial financial outlay, such as purchasing a cycle helmet or blood pressure monitoring kit, the cost may well operate as a perceived barrier affecting readiness to act. However, if researchers are to use the Health Belief Model correctly, in such an instance cost should be operationalized as a Time 1 predictor only if it is found to be among the salient psychological beliefs identified in the modal belief survey.

The research investigation we report in this chapter avoids many of the difficulties we have outlined by using Rosenstock's (1966) original disease avoidance model with its emphasis on subjective beliefs as determinants of action. The questionnaire items address perceived severity, vulnerability, benefits, barriers, and cues to action. According to the model the likelihood of cyclists adopting the preventive measure of wearing a safety helmet can be assessed by measuring their beliefs on each of the dimensions. Thus if cyclists feel sufficiently vulnerable to any number of undesirable outcomes when not wearing a helmet (such as injury, peer pressure, or parental concern), and the consequences of non-use are recognized as sufficiently severe, then the readiness to act engendered by these perceptions of threat should motivate them to evaluate the benefits and costs of wearing a helmet. This in turn will determine behaviour. In the study that follows we test both the original Rosenstock model and an expanded version in which we hypothesize that three additional variables, health locus of control (Wallston and Wallston, 1987), past behaviour (Allen and Taylor, 1984), and the subject's age, will increase explanatory power.

The Multidimensional Health Locus of Control Scale

The Multidimensional Health Locus of Control Scale (MHLC) was developed by Wallston, Wallston and DeVellis (1987). The MHLC characterizes people as perceiving the outcomes of their health behaviour to be under internal control, the control of powerful others, or the influence of chance. Several studies have found associations between health locus of control and health related behaviour (Alagna and Reddy, 1984; Hallal, 1982; McCallum et al., 1988; Muhlenkamp, Brown and Sands, 1985; Nemcek, 1990). The MHLC was thought to be an especially appropriate measure for our research since the scales can be operationalized to deal with a variety of possible influences on young cyclists. The experimental subjects, who were adolescents, may well believe that they themselves, as well as the outcomes of their behaviour, are controlled by a mixture of their own intent and the influence of significant others such as parents and teachers. Furthermore, since cycling is an activity subject to a variety of chance factors (weather conditions and road surfaces, for example) as well as personal skill, there is also scope to feel controlled by chance if an individual has that propensity. According to the theory, cyclists with an internal health locus of control should be motivated to exercise their control in response to the health threat of potential head injury by wearing a helmet; those who believe the control to rest with powerful others may wear a helmet if influenced by the advice of parents, teachers, or friends, and/or if the outcome of cycling is seen to be influenced by other road users. Cyclists with a chance health locus of control will probably be fatalistic and poorly motivated to take any constructive action.

Past behaviour

A measure of past behaviour was included in the questionnaire, since many studies have found past behaviour to be a significant influence on subsequent health behaviour (Hill, Gardner and Rassaby, 1985; Rutter, Quine and Chesham, 1990; and Sutton, in this volume). Past behaviour refers to subjects' prior experience of using the preventive measures in question, and we hypothesized that wearing a safety helmet at Time 1 would be associated with wearing a safety helmet at Time 2.

Design and method

The first stage of our work was to conduct a pilot study to explore cyclists' beliefs about wearing a helmet. Thirty schoolboys aged between eleven and eighteen who regularly cycled to school were asked about the advantages and disadvantages of wearing a helmet. This provided a set of modal beliefs for use in the main study. For the main study, a prospective design was used in which information about respondents' beliefs was obtained by a questionnaire at Time 1 and was used to predict behaviour measured four weeks later at Time 2. Subjects for the main experiment were 105 schoolboys aged between eleven and eighteen years who regularly cycled to school. They were drawn from six secondary and grammar schools in four different population centres, and so provided a representative sample of urban, semi-rural, and rural cycling conditions. Names and ages of respondents were collected to enable us to match up the Time 1 and Time 2 questionnaires. Subjects completed the first questionnaire during school hours in single sessions in a room allocated for that use. Each session began with a brief explanation of the questionnaire format and an assurance that all information was confidential. Completed questionnaires were left face down on the desks for collection by the experimenter. Four weeks later the procedure was repeated for the second questionnaire, after which the purpose of the study was explained and subjects were debriefed.

The questionnaires

Two questionnaire booklets were designed based on information gathered from the modal beliefs survey. The first booklet contained the items relating to the Health Belief Model dimensions (perceived vulnerability, severity, benefits and barriers) and the Multidimensional Health Locus of Control Scales, followed by the Time 1 behaviour items. The second booklet contained the Time 2 behaviour measure, followed by the two 'cues to action'. All behaviour items at both Time 1 and Time 2 were represented as simple yes/no questions since we had established during the pilot study that wearing a helmet was an 'all or nothing' behaviour: cyclists either wore a helmet all the time while cycling or not at all. Perceived vulnerability was measured by ten items, which asked cyclists how much more at risk of an accident they believed themselves to be than other cyclists, car drivers, and pedestrians, and how vulnerable cyclists were to slippery roads, other vehicles, and so on. Five point scales were used from 1 'strongly disagree' to 5 'strongly agree'. Perceived severity was measured by four items designed to tap how serious an effect an accident involving head injury and hospital treatment would have with respect to the cyclist's school, family, social, and personal life. Again five point scales were used, this time from 1 'very little' to 5 'very much'. There were five items for perceived benefits, e.g. 'In the event of an accident a helmet would protect my head', and five for perceived barriers, e.g. 'The colour and shape of helmets makes me look silly'. Again five point scales were used, from 1 'strongly disagree' to 5 'strongly agree'. Cues to action were measured by asking if either the subject or someone he knew well had had a cycle accident/spill in the previous four weeks. There were five items each for powerful others, internal, and chance health locus of control, adapted from Wallston, Wallston, Smith and Dobbins (1987) and Rutter et al. (1990).

The data were analysed by multiple regression, with helmet wearing the dependent variable. Though the dependent variable in multiple regression should usually be a normally distributed interval variable, regression is a robust technique and dichotomous variables may be used so long as no one category contains fewer than 20 per cent of the cases (Hedderson, 1987). The 20 per cent criterion was met in the present data, and multiple regression was therefore appropriate.

Findings

Ninety-seven cyclists answered both the Time 1 questionnaire and the Time 2 questionnaire, a response rate of 92 per cent. Average age was 13 years and 8 months, and 74.3 per cent of subjects were aged 12 to 15. At Time 2, 46 (47 per cent) were helmet users, and 51 (53 per cent) were non-users. As a first step, scales were constructed of all the major dimensions we were to use, and their reliabilities were investigated by Cronbach's alpha. Satisfactory alphas were found for all dimensions, ranging from 0.76 to 0.62.

Differences between helmet users and non-users

To test for differences in beliefs between helmet users and non-users t-tests were carried out. Table 6.1 shows that there were significant differences between means for three of the measures of the Health Belief Model and one component of the Multidimensional Health Locus of Control Scale. Helmet users were significantly more likely than non-users to believe themselves vulnerable to accidents, and were more likely than non-users to perceive the benefits of wearing a helmet but less likely to perceive the barriers. They were also significantly more likely than non-users to believe that powerful others might play a role in their safety on the road.

To investigate whether having had an accident/spill or knowing someone who had had an accident/spill in the four weeks up to the measurement of behaviour at Time 2 could act as a cue to action, we carried out Chi^2 tests. Table 6.2 shows that of those who had experienced an accident/spill themselves, 74 per cent wore a helmet at Time 2, while only 32 per cent of those who had not had an accident did so, a highly significant difference. Knowing someone who had had an accident/spill had no effect. In a third cross-tabulation we found a significant relationship between helmet use and past behaviour: of cyclists who wore a helmet at Time 1, 100 per cent wore one at Time 2, while of those who did not wear a helmet at Time 1, only 19 per cent wore one at Time 2.

Finally in this first section of results we carried out t-tests to investigate the differences in means between helmet users and non-users for each benefit and barrier separately. This gave an indication of which were the most important benefits and barriers. There were significant differences

Table 6.1
Differences between helmet users and non-users

	Helmet users (N = 46)		Non-users (N = 51)		
	Mean	s.d.	Mean	s.d.	t
Vulnerability	31.4	3.2	28.7	3.8	3.6 ***
Severity	15.2	3.4	14.0	3.6	1.7
Barriers	11.6	3.4	15.5	2.9	−6.1 ***
Benefits	20.3	2.2	16.9	3.2	6.0 ***
Internal Health Locus of Control	15.4	3.0	15.4	2.9	0.0
Powerful Others Health Locus of Control	17.8	2.5	16.2	3.1	2.8 **
Chance Health Locus of Control	14.8	3.3	14.2	3.1	1.0

** $p < 0.01$ *** $p < 0.001$

Table 6.2
Percentage of cyclists wearing a helmet at Time 2 by cues to action and past behaviour

	Chi^2	Grouping	% wearing a helmet at Time 2
Cue to action (Own accident)	15.8 ***	Had experienced an accident	74
		Had not experienced an accident	32
Cue to action (Accident of someone close)	0.3	Someone close had experienced an accident	50
		No one close had experienced an accident	45
Past behaviour (Wore helmet at Time 1)	58.0 ***	Wore helmet at Time 1	100
		Did not wear helmet at Time 1	19

*** $p < 0.001$

between helmet wearers and non-wearers for every single benefit and barrier item. Table 6.3 shows that the greatest differences were for Benefit 1 ('Wearing a helmet while cycling makes me feel safer'), Benefit 2 ('Parents worry less if I wear a helmet while cycling'), and Benefit 4 ('Wearing a helmet makes me more aware of the dangers of cycling'); and for Barrier 1 ('The colour and shape of helmets makes me look silly'), Barrier 2 ('Wearing a helmet would make me look silly if no-one else wore one'), and Barrier 3 ('The cost of buying a helmet would affect whether I wore one or not').

Correlations between predictors

The next step in our analysis was to examine the relationships between the components of the Health Belief Model and the Multidimensional Health Locus of Control Scale, by correlation. Table 6.4 shows the significant results. The correlation between perceived benefits and barriers indicates a significant negative association, which we would expect. The most significant positive correlation occurs between perceived benefits and powerful others, and perceived benefits also correlated with perceived vulnerability. These positive relationships suggest that subjects who believe in the benefits of helmet wearing are also those who perceive themselves to be vulnerable to accidents and feel influenced by the advice and actions of powerful others. There were significant positive correlations too between powerful others and both vulnerability and internal control. These indicate that cyclists who believe their behaviour to be influenced by powerful others also feel vulnerable to accidents and/or injury, as well as believing the outcomes of their cycling behaviour to be subject to their own internal control. Those cyclists who believe they can avoid accidents by cycling safely are also aware that they are subject to the vagaries of other road users.

Predicting helmet use

The last stage of our analysis was to try to predict helmet use from the Health Belief Model components (vulnerability, severity, benefits, barriers, and cues to action) and from the expanded model containing the Health Belief Model components, the Multidimensional Health Locus of Control Scale, the measure of past behaviour, and the subject's age. The technique we used was hierarchical multiple regression. Two regression analyses were performed. In the first, only the Health Belief Model components were entered: vulnerability and severity in an initial block, followed by benefits, barriers, and cues to action in a second block, as suggested by

Table 6.3
Differences between helmet users and non-users on each benefit and barrier

	Helmet users (N = 46)		Non-users (N = 51)		
	Mean	s.d.	Mean	s.d.	t
Benefit 1 Wearing a helmet while cycling makes me feel safer	4.4	0.6	3.4	1.1	6.0 ***
Benefit 2 Parents worry less if I wear a helmet while cycling	4.3	0.9	3.6	1.0	3.7 ***
Benefit 3 In the event of an accident a helmet would protect my head	4.7	0.5	4.3	0.9	2.5 *
Benefit 4 Wearing a helmet makes me more aware of the dangers of cycling	3.6	1.0	2.9	1.0	3.3 **
Benefit 5 Wearing a helmet makes me more likely to take care	3.6	1.0	2.7	1.2	3.1 **
Barrier 1 The colour and shape of helmets makes me look silly	2.7	1.3	3.8	1.0	−4.4 ***
Barrier 2 Wearing a helmet would make me look silly if no one else wore one	2.9	1.4	3.8	1.1	−3.7 ***
Barrier 3 The cost of buying a helmet would affect whether I wore one or not	2.7	1.3	3.7	1.1	−3.9 ***
Barrier 4 I do not go fast enough on my bike to need head protection in a crash	1.5	0.9	2.1	1.1	−2.6 *
Barrier 5 Wearing a helmet would not protect me in an accident	1.7	1.0	2.1	1.2	−2.1 *

* $p < 0.05$ ** $p < 0.01$ *** $p < 0.001$

Table 6.4
Significant correlations between and within the Health Belief Model variables and the Multidimensional Health Locus of Control Scale

	Vulnerability	Benefits	Barriers	Internal Health Locus of Control
Vulnerability				
Benefits	0.28 **			
Barriers	—	-0.36 **		
Internal Health Locus of Control	—	—	—	
Powerful Others Health Locus of Control	0.22 *	0.36 **	—	0.29 **

* $p < 0.05$ ** $p < 0.01$

Rosenstock (1966). The combined variables explained 53 per cent of the variance in helmet use at Time 2. Table 6.5 shows the betas for the five significant predictors: barriers (negatively); having had an accident in the previous four weeks; benefits; vulnerability; and knowing someone else who had had an accident in the previous four weeks. Only perceived severity was not significant.

In the second analysis both the Health Belief Model components and the components of our 'expanded model' were entered. Vulnerability and severity were entered first, followed by benefits, barriers, and cues to action. Then, in order to test the sufficiency of the model by examining whether the additional variables would explain a further amount of variance, the three dimensions of the Multidimensional Health Locus of Control Scale were entered, together with the measure of past behaviour and the subject's age. Table 6.6 shows that the expanded model explained 69.9 per cent of the variance in helmet use at Time 2. Vulnerability and severity explained 12.2 per cent of the variance; benefits, barriers, having had an accident, and knowing someone else who had had an accident increased the variance to 52.6 per cent; and finally, when age, and powerful others, internal, and chance health locus of control were added, together with past behaviour, the variance explained rose to 69.9 per cent. The increases between blocks were highly significant, and the third block added over 17 per cent to the variance explained, confirming the additional power of the expanded model over the HBM. Four variables made a significant contribution in the final equation: benefits, barriers, having had an accident in the previous four weeks, and past behaviour.

Discussion

Our study set out to use the Health Belief Model in a prospective design to determine whether helmet wearing in young cyclists could be predicted from health beliefs and whether the variance explained could be increased by the addition of the Multidimensional Health Locus of Control Scale, past behaviour, and the subject's age. The results provide strong support for both models. The five components of the Health Belief Model — perceived vulnerability, severity, benefits and barriers, and cues to action (the two accident measures at Time 2) — accounted for 53 per cent of variance in behaviour in the first analysis, and the components of the expanded model (five HBM dimensions, three components of the MHLC scale, past behaviour, and subject's age) accounted for almost 70 per cent of the variance in the second analysis. The findings provide strong

Table 6.5
Hierarchical multiple regression analysis of helmet use (Health Belief Model)

	Adjusted R^2	F change	Beta in Final Equation
Vulnerability			0.20 **
Severity			0.03
Block 1	11.8	—	
Benefits			0.27 ***
Barriers			−0.38 ***
Own accident			0.36 ***
Other's accident			0.17 *
Block 2	53.0	20.5 ***	

Final F = 18.1 *** df = 6

* $p < 0.05$ ** $p < 0.01$ *** $p < 0.001$

Table 6.6
Hierarchical multiple regression analysis of helmet use (expanded model)

	Adjusted R^2	F change	Beta in Final Equation
Vulnerability			0.08
Severity			−0.01
Block 1	12.2	—	
Benefits			0.15 *
Barriers			−0.17 *
Own accident			0.27 ***
Other's accident			−0.10
Block 2	52.6	19.7 ***	
Age			−0.08
Powerful others			0.03
Internal			0.02
Chance			0.05
Past behaviour			0.52 ***
Block 3	69.9	10.8 ***	

Final F = 20.1 *** df = 11

* $p < 0.05$ *** $p < 0.001$

support for the Health Belief Model and its underlying premise, that preventive health behaviour can be predicted from health beliefs.

Health Belief Model dimensions

In the first regression analysis, perceived barriers, benefits, and vulnerability (in descending order of statistical significance) were associated with helmet wearing at Time 2, while there was no association with perceived severity. This 'rank order' of dimensions is identical to that given by Janz and Becker (1984) in their review of the post-1974 HBM literature, and has also been reported by Champion (1984, 1985) and Hill et al. (1985), and more recently by Nemcek (1990), Reid and Christensen (1988), Wilson, Manual and Lavelle (1991), and Wyper (1990). In our second analysis too, barriers were the most reliable predictor, and many other studies have found the same (see Champion, 1984, 1985, 1987, 1988; Hill et al., 1985; McCallum et al, 1988; Mullen et al., 1987; Rutledge, 1987; Reid and Christensen, 1988; Hennig and Knowles, 1990; Nemcek, 1990; Oldridge and Streiner, 1990; Wyper, 1990; Aspinwall, Kemeny, Taylor, Schneider and Dudley, 1991; Clarke et al., 1991; Wilson et al., 1991).

The significance of the perceived barriers dimension may reflect its multi-dimensional nature. Champion (1984), Hill et al. (1985), Clarke et al. (1991), Hennig and Knowles (1990), and Simon, Morse, Balson, Osofsky and Gaumer (1993) all found barriers to be a multi-dimensional concept. Our own modal belief survey indicated that barriers to helmet use included doubts about the efficacy of the helmets, misconceptions about the risks associated with cycling, the cost of buying a helmet, and above all, adolescent concerns with image and identity. While all these issues would seem to militate against helmet use, the last two concerns were of particular importance, for many cyclists gave their reasons for not wearing a helmet as the adverse effects on their 'street credibility'. Specific concerns were the design and appearance of the helmets themselves, and not wanting to be the 'odd one out' by wearing one. Cost was also a factor. With all these drawbacks to helmet use it is hardly surprising that the perceived barriers dimension was found to be so significant an influence and such a good indicator of non-use. Our analysis of the data provided empirical support for the influence of these concerns, since two of the most important barriers to helmet use related to appearance. Our results reinforce the importance of conducting a preliminary survey to find out about salient beliefs in one's particular population (see Hecker and Ajzen, 1983).

The analysis of *individual barriers* provides strong support for our hypothesis that helmet users and non-users would have different sets of beliefs. The five barriers to action were subscribed to more (in terms of mean scores) by non-users than by users. The colour and shape of helmets and being conspicuous if wearing one appear to have put many cyclists off wearing a helmet, and the cost of buying a helmet was also a consideration that featured as a salient barrier among non-users. Our analysis of the separate barriers (and benefits) also supports Rosenstock's (1966) contention that the decision to undertake a course of action (or not to) follows a process of weighing up the perceived costs and benefits. Helmet users and non-users alike appear to regard the design and cost of helmets as a disadvantage. However, it seems that potential barriers do not always translate into behaviour, since a belief in the overall benefits of wearing helmets outweighs such considerations for helmet users: helmet users score significantly higher than non-users on each of the benefits items. Thus design and expense appear to become less decisive factors if a cyclist is motivated by other more salient beliefs about benefits. Our results cast doubt on the utility of promotional campaigns that attempt to encourage helmet use by reducing cost alone: the impact of helmet use on a cyclist's image, appearance and identity also need to be considered, for they too have emerged as significant influences in our study.

Perceived *benefits*, the second most important predictor of outcome behaviour, was also a multi-dimensional concern reflecting a real belief in the various benefits afforded by helmet-wearing. Of particular importance were two issues: parents worrying less, and a desire to be seen taking responsibility for personal safety. Also important was the benefit of being made more aware of the dangers of cycling. All three beliefs were subscribed to significantly more by helmet users than non-users. The belief in the protective ability of the helmets themselves was, surprisingly, accepted by both groups. That non-users believe helmets to be effective and yet do not wear them again indicates that the decision to wear or not to wear a helmet cannot be traced to any one single belief. Instead, helmet-users and non-users appear to have certain beliefs in common, and are distinguishable only by different clusters or combinations of beliefs.

By identifying the influence of *individual benefits*, we were also able to point to what were the most salient anxieties. In keeping with Rosenstock's (1966) theory, the most salient beliefs about benefits ought to reflect specific aspects of perceived vulnerability since a chosen course of action aims to reduce them. The benefits of making the cyclist feel safer and making parents worry less reduce both the personal threat and the anxieties of important others, both of which contribute to a cyclist's overall perceptions of vulnerability. There is also an indication that the benefits scale can be used to assess normative influences if these appear to be salient. Calnan and Rutter (1986) and Hecker and Ajzen (1983) have both criticized the HBM for its apparent neglect of normative beliefs. We too have now found that one of the most salient benefits in our study relates to the influence of referent others.

The relationship between *benefits and the 'powerful others' component* of the MHLC scale also reflects our concerns about normative pressure since it implies that the benefits of helmet use are partly associated with the advice and influence of others. As well as proving significant in the regression equations, benefits correlated positively with helmet use and with the cue to action, personal accidents. More importantly, benefits also correlated positively with perceived vulnerability, which indicates that helmet users feel vulnerable to the health threat implicit in road traffic accidents and believe in the value of safety helmets as a preventive measure. Both findings strongly support Rosenstock's (1966) hypothesis that a perceived threat to health provides the motive force (readiness to act) to assess and undertake an effective course of preventive action. Thus a combination of benefits and vulnerability would seem essential prerequisites for preventive health behaviour. Lindsay-Reid and Osbourne (1980) comment that within the HBM the perceptions of vulnerability to a specific health threat and the value of a health action in reducing that threat (the benefits of action) are logically related (p. 140). However, they also suggest that the relationship is likely to be strongest within the context of a single-cause disorder where the threat to health and the corresponding action are clearly related (p. 145). The threat to health of head injury as a result of a cycling accident can be viewed as just such a single-cause disorder, and one to which the benefits of wearing a helmet are clearly related. This may explain the strong association between perceived benefits and vulnerability, and also why perceived benefits were so strongly related to helmet-wearing. In studies where the benefits dimension has been a non-significant influence (Champion, 1984, 1988, 1993; Reid and Christensen, 1988; Hennig and Knowles, 1990; Nemcek, 1990; Oldridge and Streiner, 1990; Kelly et al., 1991) the health threat has often been a disorder with multiple causes, such as coronary heart disease, cancer, or stress, and the preventive action has not been readily related to the threat.

The third most significant consideration for helmet users, behind perceived barriers and perceived benefits, was perceived *vulnerability*. The strong implication is that helmet users do feel vulnerable when cycling, particularly to the risk of sustaining head injury. As well as being related to perceived benefits, vulnerability was also correlated with the powerful others locus of control scale, which refers both to referent others and to other road users. The association can be interpreted in two ways. The first is that it may indicate that referent others (parents, teachers, and road safety experts) through their actions and advice influence feelings of vulnerability in the cyclists. If this is the case, we might suggest that promotional campaigns could use such people to make cyclists more aware of their vulnerability. The second interpretation is that cyclists feel vulnerable because they are especially aware of other road users and perhaps attribute their accidents to them. We can see from the correlation between vulnerability and the 'risk-no risk' self rating that as cyclists feel more vulnerable they take fewer risks, but this might imply risks from their own cycling as much as the risk posed by other road users.

Perceived *severity*, finally, was found to be less important than the other dimensions of the HBM and was associated significantly with helmet use in only one set of correlations. This is consistent with other studies (e.g. Alagna and Reddy, 1984; Champion, 1984; Rutledge, 1987; Nemcek, 1990; Champion and Miller, 1992). Janz and Becker (1984) suggest that severity may be of minor importance in preventive health behaviour since people will seriously consider the relative severity of an illness or health outcome only when they actually have, or believe they have, an illness. Studies in which perceived severity is a significant issue do tend to be those concerning sick-role behaviour rather than preventive health behaviour (e.g. Kegeles and Lund, 1984; Oldridge and Streiner, 1990)

Non-attitudinal variables

The three non-attitudinal variables — 'past behaviour' and the two 'cues to action' — were associated significantly with helmet use in both regression analyses. Rosenstock (1974) and King (1982) propose that cues to action often differentiate between subjects who hold the relevant health beliefs and take preventive action and those who hold the same beliefs yet do nothing. The reason why having an accident was such an influential cue in our sample may be that it was an immediate and often painful experience for many of the cyclists, and one that acted as an internal cue rather than a weaker external prompt concerning a threat to health yet to be experienced. Similarly, King (1982), Calnan (1984), and Jones, Jones and Katz (1991) suggest that the presence of symptoms among their subjects acted as (internal) cues, and in Calnan's study were associated with definite feelings of vulnerability. It is reasonable to assume that having had an accident increased cyclists' awareness of their vulnerability (to head injury) and caused them to consider the benefits of safety helmets. An appreciation of the benefits in turn outweighed the salience of perceived barriers. The interaction between cues to action, perceived vulnerability, and benefits is central to the HBM.

Knowing someone who had had an accident was also a significant predictor of helmet wearing, for cues such as this may act as threat-evoking information and may influence cyclists in the same way as personal accidents. The findings suggest that an intervention based on the HBM and aimed at increasing helmet wearing could successfully invoke the motivating effects of emotional arousal. Champion and Miller (1992), investigating variables related to breast self-examination, comment that 'Having recently heard about breast cancer seemed to stimulate concurrent behaviour' (p. 93) — though there was no such effect for attendance at mammography in Vaile, Calnan, Rutter and Wall (1993). Haefner and Kirscht (1970) found that a fear-arousing message increased both feelings of vulnerability to specified illness and perceptions of the benefits of advocated preventive actions.

Finally, the past behaviour of wearing a helmet at Time 1 was also a significant factor in the regression analysis. Many researchers have found past behaviour to be important (see King, 1982; Mullen et al., 1987). Both Calnan and Rutter (1986) and Clarke et al. (1991), for example, found that previous breast self-examination practice was a major predictor of Time 2 behaviour a year later. The literature is reviewed in detail in this volume, by Sutton.

Health locus of control

The MHLC scale provided some interesting results, although contrary to expectations internality was found not to be associated with helmet use, while belief in the importance of powerful others was. This is consistent with the findings of Alagna and Reddy (1982), Hallal (1982), Muhlenkamp et al. (1985), and Nemcek (1990), who all found belief in powerful others to be associated with outcome behaviour. Kristiansen (1987) suggests that general expectancies, as measured by the MHLC scale, may influence behaviour only in novel situations (p. 75), and it may well be that internal control is associated more with prior and even habitual behaviour. McCallum et al. (1988), for example, found that internal control was associated with compliant behaviour only in subjects with prior experience of the specific behaviour under study. King (1982), Calnan (1984), and Calnan and Moss (1984) — working on screening — used measures of perceived control which corresponded to internal health locus of control. In keeping with McCallum et al. (1988), they all found that subjects who believed themselves to be in control were those most likely to have attended preventive screening services in the past. For many cyclists, however, wearing a helmet is in contrast a relatively novel experience, which from Kristiansen's (1987) point of view would seem to support the use of the MHLC scale. Even among cyclists who consistently wear a helmet, helmet use may be less attributable to habit than is the case for other preventive health behaviours. Attending a screening clinic or adhering to a diet, for example, are behaviours that are unlikely to run counter to social norms. Wearing a cycle helmet, however, is a minority practice and one that may need to be constantly re-evaluated by each individual with reference to his belief structure.

Conclusion

In summary, we have been able to predict the use of cycle safety helmets by schoolboys cycling to school, using the HBM and an expanded model. Our findings support the HBM as an effective framework for investigating preventive health behaviours, and indicate that it can be adapted to a variety of settings by the addition of measures appropriate to the behaviour being investigated and to the characteristics of the population being sampled. In the present instance the MHLC scale also appears to have been particularly well suited for use with teenagers. Adapting the model to the demands of the situation would appear more 'ecologically valid' than devising a standardized expanded model utilizing a preset questionnaire.

The findings have important implications for programmes designed to increase helmet use, since a constellation of beliefs associated with the wearing of cycle helmets has been identified that could form the basis of promotional campaigns. If a cyclist believes himself to be vulnerable to the health threat implicit in cycling (head injury), and believes that wearing a helmet would be beneficial in reducing that threat, then through the influence of referent others and the cue of having had an accident already he will probably begin to wear a helmet. Conversely, if the (psychological) costs associated with helmet use are sufficiently salient to outweigh any perceived benefits, it is unlikely that a cyclist will wear a helmet even if he feels personally vulnerable. An important role for health educators and promoters is thus to make salient the threat of injury and the benefits of action and to minimize the perceived significance of costs. The greatest success is likely to occur in the presence of perceived powerful others and salient cues to action, particularly the experience of a recent accident.

References

Ajzen, I. (1988), *Attitudes, Personality and Behavior*, Open University Press, Milton Keynes.

Alagna, S.W. and Reddy, D.M. (1984), 'Predictors of proficient technique and successful lesion detection in breast self-examination', *Health Psychology*, 3, pp. 113-27.

Allen, H.M. and Taylor, S.E. (1984), 'Alternative theories of health policy attitudes and protective behaviours: self-interest, sociotrophy and socialization', *Basic and Applied Social Psychology*, 5, pp. 19-35.

Aspinwall, L.K., Kemeny, M.E., Taylor, S.E., Schneider, S.G. and Dudley, J.P. (1991), 'Psychosocial factors of gay men's AIDS risk-reduction behaviour', *Health Psychology*, 10, pp. 432-44.

Atkinson, J.W. and Feather, N.T. (1966), *A Theory of Achievement Motivation*, Wiley, New York.

Becker, M.H. (1974), 'The Health Belief Model and sick-role behaviour', *Health Education Monographs*, 2, pp. 409-20.

Becker, M.H., Drachman, R.H. and Kirscht, J.P. (1972a), 'Predicting mothers' compliance with pediatric medical regimens', *Medical Care*, 81, pp. 843-54.

Becker, M.H., Drachman, R.H. and Kirscht, J.P. (1972b) 'Motivations as predictors of health behaviour', *Health Services Reports*, 87, pp. 852-62.

Becker, M.H., Drachman, R.H. and Kirscht, J.P. (1974), 'A new approach to explaining sick-role behaviour in low-income populations', *American Journal of Public Health*, 64, pp. 204-16.

Becker, M.H., Haefner, D.P., Kasl, S.V., Kirscht, J.P., Maiman, L.A. and Rosenstock, I.M. (1977), 'Selected psychosocial models and correlates of individual health-related behaviours', *Medical Care*, 15 (5 supplement), pp. 27-46.

Becker, M.H. and Maiman, L.A. (1975), 'Sociobehavioural determinants of compliance with health and medical care recommendations', *Medical Care*, 13, pp. 10-24.

Becker, M.H., Maiman, L.A., Kirscht, J.P., Haefner, D.P., and Drachman, R.H. (1977), 'The Health Belief Model and prediction of dietary compliance: a field experiment', *Journal of Health and Social Behaviour*, 18, pp. 348-66.

Budd, R.J., North, D. and Spencer, C. (1984), 'Understanding seat belt use: a test of Bentler and Speckart's extension of the "Theory of Reasoned Action"', *European Journal of Social Psychology*, 14, pp. 69-78.

Budd, R.J. and Spencer, C.P. (1986), 'Lay theories of behavioural intention: a source of response bias in the Theory of Reasoned Action?', *British Journal of Social Psychology*, 25, pp. 109-17.

Calnan, M. (1984), 'The Health Belief Model and participation in programmes for the early detection of breast cancer: a comparative analysis', *Social Science and Medicine*, 19, pp. 823-30.

Calnan, M. and Moss, S. (1984), 'The Health Belief Model and compliance with education given at a class in breast self-examination', *Journal of Health and Social Behaviour*, 25, pp. 198-210.

Calnan, M. and Rutter, D.R. (1986), 'Do health beliefs predict health behaviour? An analysis of breast self-examination', *Social Science and Medicine*, 22, pp. 673-8.

Champion, V.L. (1984), 'Instrument development for Health Belief Model constructs', *Advances in Nursing Science*, 6, pp. 73-85.

Champion, V.L. (1985), 'Use of the Health Belief Model in determining frequency of breast self-examination', *Research in Nursing and Health*, 8, pp. 373-9.

Champion, V.L. (1987), 'The relationship of breast self-examination to Health Belief Model variables', *Research in Nursing and Health*, 10, pp. 375-82.

Champion, V.L. (1988), 'Attitudinal variables related to intention, frequency and proficiency of breast self-examination in women 35 and over', *Research in Nursing and Health*, 11, pp. 283-91.

Champion, V.L. (1993), 'Instrument refinement for breast cancer screening behaviours', *Nursing Research*, 42, pp. 139-43.

Champion, V.L. and Miller, T.K. (1992), 'Variables related to breast self-examination', *Psychology of Women Quarterly*, 16, pp. 81-96.

Clarke, V., Hill, D., Rassaby, J., White, V. and Hirst, S. (1991), 'Determinants of continued breast self-examination practice in women of 40 years and over after personalised instruction', *Health Education Research*, 6, pp. 297-306.

Dorsch M., Woodward, A.J. and Somers, R.L. (1987), 'Do bicycle safety helmets reduce the severity of head injuries in real crashes?', *Accident Analysis and Prevention*, 20, pp. 447-58.

Fishbein, M. and Ajzen, I. (1975), *Belief, Attitude, Intention and Behaviour: an Introduction to Theory and Research*, Addison-Wesley, Reading, Mass.

Gielen, A.C., Ericksen, M.P., Daltoy, L.H. and Rost, K. (1984), 'Factors associated with the use of child restraint devices', *Health Education Quarterly*, 11, pp. 195-206.

Grube, J.W., Morgan, M. and McGree, S.T. (1986), 'Attitudes and normative beliefs as predictors of smoking intentions and behaviours: a test of three models', *British Journal of Social Psychology*, 25, pp. 81-93.

Haefner, D.P. and Kirscht, J.P. (1970), 'Motivational and behavioural effects of modifying health beliefs', *Public Health Reports*, 85, pp. 478-84.

Hallal, J.C. (1982), 'The relationship of health beliefs, health locus of control, and self concept to the practice of breast self-examination in adult women', *Nursing Research*, 31, pp. 137-42.
Hecker, B.K. and Ajzen, I. (1983), 'Improving the prediction of health behaviour: an approach based on the Theory of Reasoned Action', *Academic Psychology Bulletin*, 5, pp. 11-19.
Hedderson, J. (1987), *SPSS Made Simple*, Wadsworth, Belmont, CA.
Hennig, P. and Knowles, A. (1990), 'Factors influencing women over 40 years to take precautions against cervical cancer', *Journal of Applied Social Psychology*, 20, pp. 1612-21.
Hill, D., Gardner, G. and Rassaby, J. (1985), 'Factors predisposing women to take precautions against breast and cervix cancer', *Journal of Applied Social Psychology*, 15, pp. 59-79.
Janz, N.K. and Becker, M.H. (1984), 'The Health Belief Model: a decade later', *Health Education Quarterly*, 11, pp. 1-47.
Jones, D. (1989), 'Child casualties in road accidents', in Department of Transport, *Road Accidents Great Britain 1989: The Casualty Report*, HMSO, London, pp. 37-40.
Jones, S.L., Jones, P.K. and Katz, J. (1991), 'Compliance in acute and chronic patients receiving a health belief model intervention in the emergency department', *Social Science and Medicine*, 32, pp. 1183-9.
Kasl, S.V. and Cobb, S. (1966), 'Health behaviour, illness behaviour and sick-role behaviour', *Archives of Environmental Health*, 1, 12, pp. 246-66.
Kegeles, S.S. and Lund, A.K. (1984), 'Adolescent health beliefs and acceptance of a novel dental activity: a further note', *Social Science and Medicine*, 19, pp. 979-82.
Kelly, R.B., Zyzanski, S.J., and Alemagno, S.A. (1991), 'Prediction of motivation and behaviour change following health promotion: role of health beliefs, social support, and self-efficacy', *Social Science and Medicine*, 32, pp. 311-20.
King, J. (1982), 'The impact of patients' perceptions of high blood pressure on attendance at screening', *Social Science and Medicine*, 16, pp. 1079-91.
Kristiansen, C.M. (1987), 'Social learning theory and preventive health behaviour: some neglected variables', *Social Behaviour*, 2, pp. 73-86.
Lewin, K. (1935), *A Dynamic Theory of Personality*, McGraw-Hill, London.
Lindsay-Reid, E. and Osbourne, R.W. (1980), 'Readiness for exercise adoption', *Social Science and Medicine*, 14A, pp. 139-46.
McCallum, D.M., Wiebe, D.J. and Keith, B.R. (1988), 'Effects of previous medication experience and health beliefs on intended compliance to an imagined regimen', *Journal of Compliance in Health Care*, 3, pp. 125-34.

McDermot, F.T. and Klug, G.L. (1982), 'Differences in head injuries of pedal cyclist and motor cyclist casualties in Victoria', *Medical Journal of Australia*, 2, pp. 30-32.

Melnyk, K.A. (1988), 'Barriers: a critical review of recent literature', *Nursing Research*, 37, pp. 196-201.

Mills, P.J. (1989), 'Pedal cycle accidents: a hospital based study', *TRRL Research Report 220*, Transport and Road Research Laboratory, .

Muhlenkamp, A.F., Brown, N.J. and Sands, D. (1985), 'Determinants of health promotion activities in nursing clinic clients', *Nursing Research*, 34, pp. 327-32.

Mullen, P.D., Hersey, J.C. and Iverson, D.C. (1987), 'Health behaviour models compared', *Social Science and Medicine*, 24, pp. 973-81.

Nelson, G.D. and Moffit, P.B. (1988), 'Safety belt promotion: theory and practice', *Accident Analysis and Prevention*, 20, pp. 27-38.

Nemcek, M.A. (1990), 'Health beliefs and breast self-examination among black women', *Health Values, Health Behaviour, Education and Promotion*, 14 (5), pp. 41-52.

Oldridge, N.B. and Streiner, D.L. (1990), 'The Health Belief Model: predicting compliance and dropout in cardiac rehabilitation', *Medicine and Science in Sport and Exercise*, 22, pp. 678-83.

Pitt, W.R., Thomas, S., Nixon, J., Clark, R., Battistutta, D. and Acton, C. (1994), 'Trends in head injuries among child bicyclists', *British Medical Journal*, 308, pp. 177-8.

Reid, L.D. and Christensen, D.B. (1988), 'A psychological perspective in the explanation of patients' drug-taking behaviour', *Social Science and Medicine*, 27, pp. 277-85.

Rosenstock, I.M. (1960), 'What research in motivation suggests for public health', *American Journal of Public Health*, 50, pp. 295-302.

Rosenstock, I.M. (1966), 'Why people use health services', *Millbank Memorial Fund Quarterly*, 44 (supplement), pp. 94-127.

Rosenstock, I.M. (1974), 'The Health Belief Model and preventive health behaviour', *Health Education Monographs*, 2, pp. 354-86.

Rutledge, D.N. (1987), 'Factors related to women's practice of breast self-examination', *Nursing Research*, 36, pp. 117-21.

Rutter, D.R., Quine, L. and Chesham, D.J. (1990), 'Do motorcyclists' beliefs predict accident liability?', in Benjamin, T. (ed.), *Driving Behaviour in a Social Context*, Paradigme, Caen, pp. 172-180.

Rutter, D.R., Quine, L. and Chesham, D.J. (1993), *Social Psychological Approaches to Health*, Harvester Wheatsheaf, Hemel Hempstead.

Simon, P.M., Morse, E.V., Balson, P.M., Osofsky, H.J. and Gaumer, H.R. (1993), 'Barriers to human immunodeficiency virus related risk reduction

among male street prostitutes', *Health Education Quarterly*, 20, pp. 261-73.
Stasson, M. and Fishbein, M. (1990), 'The relation between perceived risk and preventive action: a within-subjects analysis of perceived driving risk and intentions to wear seatbelts', *Journal of Applied Social Psychology*, 20, pp. 1541-57.
Stutts, J.C., Williamson, J.E., Whitley, T. and Sheldon, F.C. (1990), 'Bicycle accidents and injuries: a pilot study comparing hospital- and police-reported data', *Accident Analysis and Prevention*, 22, pp. 67-78.
Sutton, S. and Hallett, R. (1989), 'Understanding seat-belt intentions and behavior: a decision-making approach', *Journal of Applied Social Psychology*, 19, pp. 1310-25.
Taylor, S. (1989), 'Pedal cycle casualties', in Department of Transport, *Road Accidents Great Britain 1989: The Casualty Report*, HMSO, London, pp. 41-6.
Thomas, S., Acton, C., Nixon, J., Battistutta, D., Pitt, W.R. and Clark, R. (1994), 'Effectiveness of bicycle helmets in preventing head injury in children: case-control study', *British Medical Journal*, 308, pp. 173-6.
Vaile, M.S.B., Calnan, M., Rutter, D.R. and Wall, B. (1993), 'Breast cancer screening services in three areas: uptake and satisfaction', *Journal of Public Health Medicine*, 15, pp. 37-45.
Wallston, K.A., Wallston, B.S. and DeVellis, R. (1987), 'Development of the Multidimensional Health Locus of Control (MHLC) scales', *Health Education Monographs*, 6, pp. 160-70.
Wallston, K.A., Wallston, B.S., Smith, M.S. and Dobbins, C.J. (1987), 'Perceived control and health', *Current Psychology Research and Reviews*, 6, pp. 5-25.
Webb, G.R., Sanson-Fisher, R.W. and Bowman, J.A. (1988), 'Psychosocial factors related to parental restraint of pre-school children in motor vehicles', *Accident Analysis and Prevention*, 20, pp. 97-94.
Williams, M. (1990), 'Evaluation of the penetration test for bicylists' helmets: comparative performance of hard shell and foam helmets', *Accident Analysis and Prevention*, 22, pp. 315-25.
Williams, M. (1991), 'The protective performance of bicyclists' helmets in accidents', *Accident Analysis and Prevention*, 23, pp. 119-31.
Wilson, D., Manual, A. and Lavelle, S. (1991), 'Psychological predictors of condom use to prevent HIV transmission among Zimbabwean students', *International Journal of Psychology*, 26, pp. 705-21.
Wittenbraker, J., Gibbs, B.L. and Kahle, L.R. (1983), 'Seat belt attitudes, habits, and behaviors: an adaptive amendment to the Fishbein model', *Journal of Applied Social Psychology*, 13, pp. 406-421.

Wood, T. and Milne, P. (1988), 'Head injuries to pedal cyclists and the promotion of helmet use in Victoria, Australia', *Accident Analysis and Prevention*, 20, pp. 177-85.
Wyper, M.A. (1990), 'Breast self-examination and the Health Belief Model: variations on a theme', *Research in Nursing and Health*, 13, pp. 421-8.

7 Risk appraisal and health behaviour

Joop van der Pligt

This chapter summarizes a number of social psychological models that aim to describe and explain health behaviour. It will be argued that the prevailing models are all based on expectancy-value approaches to human judgement and choice. The models combine *probability* judgements (e.g. the likelihood of negative and positive health consequences of one's behaviour) and *value* judgements (the evaluation or the expected utility of the consequences). After a brief summary of the models I shall discuss one issue in more detail: the perception or appraisal of health risks and the role of positive illusions such as unrealistic optimism. In most models of health behaviour perceived risk for one's health plays an important role. Biases in risk perception, their causes, and the behavioural consequences of perceived risk will be examined. The behavioural consequences will also be discussed in the context of more general models of health behaviour.

Models of health behaviour

Fishbein and Ajzen's (1975) Theory of Reasoned Action and the more recent Theory of Planned Behaviour (Ajzen, 1985, 1991) are based on Subjective Expected Utility theory (SEU) introduced by Edwards (1954). Edwards' theory assumes that people generally aim to maximize utility and prefer behavioural options that are associated with the highest expected utility. The overall utility or desirability of a behavioural alternative is assumed to be based on the summed products of the probability and utility of specific outcomes or consequences.

Thus:

$$SEU_j = \sum_i P_{ij} . U_{ij}$$

where SEU_j is the SEU of action or behavioural alternative j, P_{ij} is the perceived probability of outcome i of action j, and U_{ij} is the subjective utility or desirability of outcome i of action j. Each action or behavioural alternative may have a different Subjective Expected Utility because of the outcomes associated with that action and/or the different probabilities of the outcomes for different actions.

SEU theory allows for a subjective assessment of probability and utility but assumes that they are combined in a rational, consistent way. For instance the choice to opt for a specific diet would be a function of the assumed probabilities of losing weight, increasing fitness, and craving for food. The overall utility of the two options (go on a diet or not) would depend on the likelihood of the various consequences and the utility or desirability of each of them.

Fishbein and Ajzen (1975) extended SEU theory and formulated their Theory of Reasoned Action. According to the theory, behavioural intentions are a function of attitudes and social norms. Attitudes are assumed to be based on the summed products of the likelihood of positive and negative consequences associated with behavioural options and the evaluation of those consequences. Thus, the more positively consequences are associated with a specific behaviour and the more likely their occurrence, the more attractive the behaviour. Attitudes are assumed to be based on a rational and relatively complete cost-benefit analysis of the various (possible) consequences of behavioural alternatives. Fishbein and Ajzen (1975) argued, however, that individual attitudes (mediated by intentions) are only one determinant of behaviour. The norms in one's immediate environment were also assumed to be important, and perceived norms about behavioural options made up a second, independent, determinant of behaviour. For instance, an individual smoker could have a negative attitude towards smoking which the majority of relevant others in his or her social environment do not share. In this case attitudes and social norms would have a divergent impact on behavioural intentions. Fishbein and Ajzen argued that it is important to assess the weight of each of the two determinants of behavioural intentions. In some domains one would expect a greater impact of individual attitudes, in others a greater impact of the norms in one's environment. Similarly, some people are more influenced by subjective (social) norms than others.

The Theory of Reasoned Action presents a coherent framework for studying behavioural choice. It has frequently been applied to health related behaviours ranging from smoking cigarettes, dieting, alcohol consumption, and wearing seatbelts, to birth control measures. Overall the model provides adequate predictions of health behaviour. The theory has received extensive empirical support (see Sheppard, Hartwick and Warshaw, 1988 for a meta-analysis), particularly for behaviours that are under complete volitional control.

Ajzen (1985, 1991) argued that many behaviours are *not* under (total) volitional control, for people could have positive attitudes towards certain behaviours but simply lack the resources to carry out the behaviour. For instance, one could have a positive attitude towards giving up smoking but fail to do so because of one's limited ability to sustain the behaviour. Ajzen incorporated the variable in his revision of the Theory of Reasoned Action and termed it 'perceived behavioural control'. Perceived behavioural control is closely related to Bandura's (1989) concept 'self-efficacy' — the subjective belief of the individual in his or her ability to carry out a specific behaviour (e.g. stopping smoking, keeping to a diet, etc.). Ajzen's model is termed the Theory of Planned Behaviour and has been applied to a variety of behaviours such as shopping (Madden, Ellen and Ajzen, 1992), food intake (Sparks, Hedderly and Shepherd, 1991) and violations of traffic regulations (Parker, Manstead, Stradling, Reason and Baxter, 1992). The theory has also been applied successfully in several health settings such as giving up smoking (De Vries, Dijkstra and Kuhlman, 1988), weight reduction (Schifter and Ajzen, 1985), and infants' sugar intake (Beale and Manstead, 1991).

Fishbein and Ajzen's models assume that attitudes towards a specific behaviour are based on five to nine model salient beliefs about possible behavioural consequences. As argued by Van der Pligt and Eiser (1984), this assumption is not, however, in accordance with results obtained in the area of cognitive psychology, where findings point to the limited information processing capabilities of human decision makers. Multiplicative rules such as those presumed by SEU theory and expectancy-value approaches are quite difficult to apply and it is unrealistic to expect that people *will* apply them, especially when there are many relevant attributes and varying probabilities associated with each of the attributes or behavioural consequences. Research using the models of Ajzen and Fishbein frequently presents respondents with twenty attributes or more, and Van der Pligt and Eiser (1984) identified studies on health behaviour which included as many as fifty. It is difficult to know what it means if one can predict behaviour on the basis of large numbers of attributes, especially if it is extremely unlikely that respondents used all of them in their decision making. Van der Pligt and Eiser argued that one should allow for individual or group differences and investigate attributes that are *important* or *salient* for specific individuals or groups. In this way one could get more insight into the *structure* of individual or group attitudes and reduce the analysis of the decision making process to manageable and more realistic proportions. Van der Pligt and Eiser also argued that attitudes can be predicted adequately from individual beliefs about three to five important consequences. The selected consequences can be quite different for different groups, however. This seems especially relevant in the context of health education if we are to prevent campaigns from focusing on consequences that are seen as less relevant by the target group. For instance, Van der Pligt and Eiser (1984) reported findings which indicated that smoking and non smoking adolescents emphasized very different consequences of smoking and non smoking. Moreover, it seemed that health education campaigns did not focus on the most salient beliefs of smokers and often provided information about consequences that were seen as less relevant by smokers than non smokers. Education campaigns that focus on consequences that are seen as important by the target group, and at the same time attempt to increase the importance of the consequences that are seen as less relevant (e.g. the long term health consequences), could well be more successful in persuading people to change their behaviour.

The framework most widely used to explain preventive health behaviours is probably the *Health Belief Model* (HBM) (see for example Kirscht, 1983; Janz and Becker, 1984; and Arnold and Quine in this volume). The HBM distinguishes five factors that influence the adoption of preventive risk reducing behavioural practices. They are (a) perceived susceptibility or vulnerability to developing a specific health problem, (b) perceived severity of that problem, (c) perceived benefits of behavioural action(s), (d) perceived barriers and/or possible negative consequences of the action(s), and (e) specific cues to action, such as symptoms, more direct experiences of the health problem in one's environment, or a health education campaign (see Janz and Becker, 1984). A person's tendency to take a preventive action is assumed to be strongest when perceived severity, susceptibility, and benefits are high, while the costs of behavioural change are low.

The Health Belief Model has been applied extensively to issues related to *preventive* health behaviour. It needs to be added, however, that the model is less specific about how to *measure* the various antecedents of health behaviour. Moreover, it does not include clear hypotheses about the relationship between the five factors and their relative weights in predicting preventive behaviour. Generally, the model has been found useful in understanding and predicting preventive health behaviour. Results have been somewhat inconsistent, however, especially concerning the role of perceived severity and susceptibility (see for example Ronis, 1992). The utility of the HBM has been questioned when dealing with relatively severe health threats (see for example Montgomery, Joseph, Becker, Ostrow, Kessler and Kirscht, 1989). A recent direct comparison of the HBM with Ajzen's model indicated the superior predictive power of the latter (Bakker, Buunk and Siero, 1994), and it has been proposed that the HBM and SEU theory should be combined in order to generate a model that is more specific in its predictions (Ronis, 1992).

Closer inspection of the Fishbein and Ajzen models and the Health Belief Model reveals considerable overlap. Perceived susceptibility, perceived severity, and the perceived benefits and costs of behavioural change are all part of the subjective cost-benefit analysis that determines individual attitudes in the models proposed by Fishbein and Ajzen. Perceived barriers are closely related to Ajzen's concept of 'perceived behavioural control'. As argued before, one reason for the seemingly superior predictive power of the models proposed by Fishbein and Ajzen could be the well established procedures to measure the relevant concepts (attitudes, social norms, and perceived control).

A variety of other models have been developed to deal with *specific* health threats. Generally, they can be redefined in terms of the three models discussed already. For instance, Fisher and Fisher (1992) proposed a model focusing on one specific domain of health behaviour (AIDS prevention). This information-motivation-behavioural skills (IMB) model focuses on three determinants of preventive action: risk reduction information, risk reduction motivation, and risk reduction behavioural skills. Closer inspection reveals that the first factor concerns knowledge about risks, the second can be redefined in terms of the attitudinal components of Fishbein and Ajzen's model, while the third refers to self-efficacy or perceived behavioural control.

All three major models discussed thus far pay only limited attention to motivation. A number of general models focus on vulnerability and risks as threatening and fear arousing variables that can lead to a variety of cognitive, emotional and behavioural responses. For instance, the fear drive model of Leventhal, Safer and Panagis (1983) is based on the assumption that fear produces discomfort and tension, which leads to action. Janis and Mann's (1977) conflict theory also describes decisions in threatening circumstances and focuses on adaptive and maladaptive coping styles. Similarly, Rogers and his associates (Rogers, 1975; Rippetoe and Rogers, 1987) introduced protection motivation theory to account for individual reactions to information about health risks. According to protection motivation theory, informational sources initiate two appraisal processes: *threat appraisal* and *coping appraisal*. The theory distinguishes maladaptive and adaptive responses and a number of factors that facilitate or inhibit the likelihood of those responses. Threat appraisal focuses on the factors associated with the response, i.e. perceived severity of the consequences of a specific behaviour and one's perceived vulnerability to the (negative) consequences, and perceived risk thus plays an important role. The coping-appraisal process refers to the ability to cope with and avert the negative consequences. The efficacy of the response (beliefs that the recommended behaviour reduces the likelihood of the consequences) and one's ability to carry out the recommended behaviour successfully (self-efficacy) should increase the likelihood of the adaptive response. Response costs, such as abstaining from behaviour that provides pleasure, decrease the probability of occurrence of the adaptive response. Threat and coping appraisal processes are expected to mediate the persuasive effects of a fear arousing health education campaign by eliciting protection motivation. Protection motivation is expected to arouse, sustain, and direct activity to cope with threat and to determine the likelihood of the adoption of risk reducing or preventive behaviour (Rippetoe and Rogers, 1987).

The major contribution of protection motivation theory is that it explicitly addresses coping processes, and hence motivational factors, in the explanation of health behaviour. Rippetoe and Rogers (1987) point to the possible role of a variety of maladaptive coping styles such as denial and fatalism. The relevance of coping styles was also acknowledged by the early work of Janis and Mann (1977), who were concerned with the implications of conflict theory in the context of threatening information, such as information about adverse health consequences. Three coping styles identified by Janis and Mann have been frequently applied to health related behaviours. *Vigilance* refers to seeking accurate and complete information, and then analysing the problem and planning behaviour to reduce or minimize the threat. *Defensive avoidance* is a strategy that is often used to reduce stress by denying threatening information or actively evading the threat. *Hypervigilance* refers to a process of panic-like searching for appropriate responses, without reaching well balanced decisions.

Theories that explicitly address the role of motivational processes seem especially relevant in the context of immediate and relatively extreme health threats. Coping styles could help our understanding of individual health behaviours, but seem less relevant in the context of long term health consequences. For instance, the fact that adolescents may ignore the health consequences of smoking can hardly be seen as a defensive coping style: for them the threat often concerns a long term risk that is simply not acknowledged in their decision making. However, models incorporating coping processes have been useful for predicting and explaining a variety of health behaviours, such as AIDS preventive measures (Van der Velde and Van der Pligt, 1991) and breast self-examination (Rippetoe and Rogers, 1987).

All in all, most models of preventive health behaviour incorporate the recognition of one's own risk status or vulnerability as an important condition for adopting behaviours that reduce those risks. Some of the more recent models, such as protection motivation theory, focus on the motivating effects of anxiety or fear triggered by threatening information about personal risks, and on adaptive versus maladaptive coping styles. In the next sections we concentrate on perceived risk, the accuracy of people's perceptions of risk, possible biases in risk perception, and the behavioural consequences of subjective risk appraisals. Risk is generally defined as a multiplicative function of the probability of the negative consequence(s) and the evaluation of the consequence(s). In the remainder of this chapter we shall use the term risk perception to refer to the *probability* component of risk.

Risk perception

Initially, research on risk perception tended to focus on large scale societal risks such as those of nuclear energy and toxic chemicals (see for example Fischhoff, Lichtenstein, Slovic, Derby and Keeney, 1981; Van der Pligt, 1992). Risk perception has also been studied for a wide variety of personal risks such as being a victim of crime (Weinstein, 1980), divorce (Perloff and Farbisz, 1985), and traffic accidents (Svenson, 1981). Quite a few studies focus on health risks (e.g. Harris and Guten, 1979; Slovic, Fischhoff, and Lichtenstein, 1978; Weinstein, 1982; Van der Velde, Hooijkaas and Van der Pligt, 1992, Otten and Van der Pligt, 1992).

A number of conclusions can be drawn from this research. First, perceptions of risk vary considerably among people and often show little correspondence with epidemiological findings or accident statistics. *Absolute*, quantitative risk judgements are prone to a number of biases. Small probabilities are overestimated, large probabilities are underestimated. Second, risks that are more 'available' due to (for example) personal experience or media coverage tend to be overestimated. The 'availability' heuristic (Tversky and Kahneman, 1974) refers to the tendency for an event to be judged more probable when it is more easily pictured or recalled. This applies especially to more 'sensational' risks. For instance, estimates of absolute risk for AIDS tend to be too high, while estimates tend to be too low for risks such as heart disease.

Research in this area suggests that quantitative risk appraisals need to be treated with caution. This is underlined by the significant influence of the response format on risk estimates: quantitative appraisals of risks tend to be relatively unstable and influenced by the way the question is asked. It needs to be added, however, that people have a reasonable idea of the *relative* risks of various technologies and behaviours. Their orderings are similar to official statistics and epidemiological findings. Major errors seem to occur primarily in their estimates of the *magnitude* of the risks.

Although people are quite aware of the *relative* risk of specific activities or behaviours, things change rather dramatically when this knowledge is applied to their own behaviour. For instance, many smokers accept the association between smoking cigarettes and disease, but do not believe themselves to be personally at risk (Pechacek and Danaher, 1979). A substantial amount of research has focused on *cognitive* biases causing erroneous risk appraisals. This work tends to stress the effects of cognitive heuristics such as the availability heuristic. In the context of more personal risks some authors stress the possible role of motivational factors. Some have argued that cognitive heuristics are used to fulfil certain needs of the individual (see for example Gladis, Michela, Walter and Vaughan, 1992). Motivational explanations of perceived *in*vulnerability tend to focus on the need to reduce feelings of fear and anxiety. Support for the role of these mechanisms is provided by research showing more biased risk estimates in situations of increased threat. Bauman and Siegel (1987) investigated the extent of defensive denial about AIDS risks in a sample of gay men. Their findings showed that men who deny or underestimate their risk of an HIV infection experience lower anxiety. On the basis of this (correlational) finding they concluded that denial is used as a strategy to manage anxiety.

Findings such as these suggest that defensive denial may occur primarily when the possible adverse consequences for one's health are immediate and serious and one has some reason for believing oneself to be at risk. Some of these adverse consequences have been investigated in the context of groups at risk from AIDS, and have included psychological distress, barriers to behavioural change, social role impairment, and more intrusive worries and concerns about AIDS (see for example Joseph, Montgomery, Emmons, Kirscht, Kessler, Ostrow, Wortman, O'Brien and Eshleman, 1987). Taylor, Kemeny, Aspinwall, Schneider, Rodriguez, and Herbert (1992) found that optimism (dispositional optimism as assessed by a series of generalized expectancies) resulted in lower feelings of distress among a group of people at risk (in this case gay and bisexual men who were at risk of developing AIDS). Gladis, Michela, Walter and Vaughan (1992) also found evidence for motivated denial of AIDS related risks among a sample of high school students. Respondents with a dispositional tendency to deny threats were found to be more likely to misperceive personal risk. Moreover, perceived absolute risk was found to be negatively correlated with the degree of behavioural risk, i.e. for those subjects more risky practices were associated with lower perceived risk.

This obviously poses a problem for health education. A direct confrontational approach could have potentially adverse consequences for those who perceive themselves to be at greater risk. The complex dual aim of health education programmes is to create and maintain a level of anxiety that is sufficient to motivate risk reducing behaviours, but which at the same time is not too high (see also Van der Pligt, Otten, Richard and Van der Velde, 1993). As argued before, absolute risk appraisals tend to be biased, and these estimates are influenced by cognitive and motivational factors as well as contextual factors such as response format. Some researchers prefer to rely on *comparative* risk appraisals; it is to these that we now turn.

Comparative risk appraisal

A substantial body of research on the perception of health risks has focused on *comparative* risks; i.e. one's own perceived risk as compared to others. When asked to compare their risk to the 'average' person or to comparable others, many more people estimate their risk of experiencing a negative event as below average than as above average. This illusion of (relative) invulnerability has been obtained for a wide variety of health risks, ranging from 'catching a cold' to more serious risks such as heart disease, cancers, and AIDS (see for example Weinstein, 1982). One could argue that unrealistic optimism and the illusion of (relative) invulnerability hinder behavioural change, i.e. the adoption and maintenance of preventive behaviours. If health risks primarily concern other people and not oneself there is no reason to adapt one's behaviour. It seems crucial therefore to understand better the possible causes of these positive illusions and to investigate their behavioural consequences. First we turn to the possible mechanisms underlying optimistic biases.

Unrealistic optimism has been related to a variety of possible causes, some of which could also affect the accuracy of absolute risk assessment. Unfortunately, most research on unrealistic optimism uses correlational designs with the usual drawbacks for conclusions about the possible causal role of specific factors. In this section I shall briefly outline six possible causes: perceived control, egocentric biases, personal experience, stereotyped beliefs about victims, self-esteem maintenance and defensive coping styles. The first four refer to cognitive mechanisms, while the remaining two stress the role of motivational processes.

Perceived control

Weinstein (1980) noted that optimism tends to increase for risks judged to be controllable by personal action. The finding is confirmed by research showing that optimism tends to be greater for those risks judged to be under personal control (Weinstein, 1982). Other findings indicate that for each specific hazard those who rate its controllability higher are also more optimistic. This relation between perceived controllability and optimism is confirmed by research on risk appraisals in the context of AIDS (Van der Velde et al. 1992).

Egocentric bias

Another factor that could be related to optimism is what Weinstein (1980) termed egocentric bias. When people are asked to assess their risks and those of others, they simply have more knowledge about their own protective actions than those of others. It seems that people tend to focus on personal actions that *reduce* their risks while they tend to forget personal actions or circumstances that *increase* their risks. Moreover, one's own actions are more available than those of others – the cognitive availability heuristic mentioned earlier (Tversky and Kahneman, 1974). That is, we have more knowledge about our own preventive actions than those of others. Weinstein (1983) showed that when college students describe their own standing on risk factors *and* are given explicit information about the risk status of their peers on those factors, optimistic biases are substantially reduced. Since the procedure had little effect on judgements for threats that do not normally evoke unrealistic optimism, Weinstein (1983) concluded that the treatment eliminated a bias and did not simply create pessimism. Thus, receiving feedback about preventive actions of others reduced egocentrism. Interestingly, asking subjects to consider their own standing on risk factors *without* providing them with information about comparable others substantially *increased* optimistic biases. It thus seems that exclusive attention to one's own risk status prevents people realizing that most others show similar behaviour.

Personal experience

Weinstein (1980, 1982) concluded that lack of previous personal experience tends to increase unrealistic optimism. Personal experience is a powerful stimulus to action (see Weinstein, 1989 for a review), tends to be concrete and relatively vivid as compared to statistical information about risks, and enhances cognitive availability. Thus, possible negative consequences for health and well-being that have been experienced more directly (oneself, close friends or relatives as victims) tend to result in less optimistic risk appraisals.

Stereotyped beliefs

Another factor that could produce unrealistic optimism is related to stereotyped judgement; i.e. a relatively extreme image of those suffering from specific diseases. An extreme prototype is unlikely to fit one's self-image, hence the idea that the risk applies primarily to others.

Self-esteem maintenance

Weinstein (1984) suggested that self-esteem maintenance or enhancement could be a major determinant of unrealistic optimism. Generally, people seem to think that their actions, lifestyle, and personality are more advantageous than those of their peers. This mechanism would explain the fact that people are *most* optimistic about controllable risks and far less so about hereditary and environmental health risks. The latter are not likely to constitute a threat to one's self-esteem. A high risk lifestyle, on the other hand, implies that we are ignorant of what we ought to do or are simply unable to exercise self-control. Both ignorance and limited ability have clear links to self-esteem. Self-esteem maintenance is also related to the previous factor (stereotyped beliefs), for both involve social comparison processes.

Defensive denial

Under conditions of high stress or threat, denial often helps to protect against anxiety and worry. There is some evidence for the role of defensive strategies. In a study in which optimism about each of forty-five different health and life threatening problems was related to characteristics of the problems, Weinstein (1982) found that more threatening health risks were associated with higher levels of optimism. On the other hand, the results also showed that increased worry about health risks was associated with *less* optimism — a finding that contradicts the obtained relationship between seriousness of consequences and optimism. Van der Velde et al. (1991, 1992) found defensive denial (as a more general coping style) to be positively related to optimism about AIDS related risks. Optimism also affected the perceived seriousness of the possible consequences and was associated with a reduced belief in one's ability to reduce the risks.

All six factors described in this section seem to play a role in the formation and maintenance of unrealistic optimism. A number of weaknesses need to be mentioned, however. First, the six factors are not mutually exclusive. It seems difficult to disentangle the various cognitive and motivational processes that could produce unrealistic optimism. The availability heuristic can explain some of the findings, and seems the most important cognitive factor underlying unrealistic optimism, but it cannot explain them all. Unrealistic optimism refers to a comparative risk assessment, suggesting that social comparison processes also play an important role. Overestimating one's personal control over specific health risks and selecting stereotyped others as potential victims could be seen as mechanisms to enhance one's self-esteem. Finally, motivational needs could also lead to optimism. The need to reduce fear and anxiety could lead to unrealistic optimism about health risks. Motivational mechanisms thus seem most likely to occur when the health risk is immediate and concerns irreversible and relatively extreme outcomes.

In summary, both cognitive and motivational factors affect risk appraisal. Generally, cognitive factors seem to provide the best explanation for biases in absolute risk appraisals. Motivational factors such as fear and anxiety reduction seem to be most relevant for relatively immediate and serious risks to one's health. Motivational factors such as self-esteem maintenance seem to be more prominent in explaining comparative risk appraisals – for example, unrealistic optimism. As Taylor and Brown (1988) argue, positive illusions such as optimism have a functional value and can improve well-being, task performance, and recovery from illness. Scheier and Carver (1992) provide an overview of the beneficial effects of optimism on psychological and physical well-being, and argue that they include improved ability to cope with stressful life events. In the context of health risks, however, optimism can sometimes be *dysfunctional*, for it can hinder the adoption and/or maintenance of preventive behaviour. It is to this issue that I shall turn in the next section, where the relation between perceived risk and behaviour will be discussed.

Perceived risk, optimism and behaviour

In this section I shall focus on the *consequences* of unrealistic optimism. The applied value of research on unrealistic optimism is that optimism could make people think they are relatively invulnerable. Perceived invulnerability, in turn, could undermine the motivation to take precautions. There is some evidence to show that perceptions of vulnerability do predict preventive health behaviour (Becker, Haefner, Kasl, Kirscht, Maiman and Rosenstock, 1977; Cummings, Jette, Brock and Haefner, 1979; Kasl, 1975). Other research, however, shows no relationship between susceptibility or perceived risk and behaviour, and sometimes even shows a relationship opposite to that predicted (see for example Gerrard, Gibbons, and Warner, 1993). The 'modest' predictive power of perceived risk seems to be greatest for serious risks. Two cautionary notes are in order, however. First, many studies have employed 'one shot' designs in which perceived risk and intentions to take preventive action are assessed at the same time. It needs to be added that prospective, longitudinal studies on AIDS preventive behaviour also show mixed findings for the predictive power of perceived risk. Unfortunately, longitudinal designs seem to be the exception rather than the rule. Second, perceived risk has been assessed in a variety of ways, ranging from numerical estimates (probability scores, annual death rates) to scores derived from verbal categories. An important (and often neglected) aspect concerns the conditional nature of perceived risk. Generally, perceived risk has been assessed in very general terms without referring to specific behaviours and/or a specific time period. It is important also to investigate the perception of risk conditional on the presence or absence of preventive action (see for example Ronis, 1992). Strictly speaking, most models require a conditional risk estimate.

Otten and Van der Pligt (1992) attempted to assess whether individual risk appraisal mediates the relation between past and future behaviour. They expected that risks associated with past behaviour would affect risk appraisal and intentions about future behaviour. To assess the mediating role of risk appraisal they investigated four separate relationships: first, the relationship between past behaviour and future behavioural intentions; second, the relationship between past behavioural practices and risk appraisal; third, the relationship between risk appraisal and behavioural intentions; and finally, the relationship between risk appraisal and behavioural intentions controlling for risk appraisal. Otten and Van der Pligt tested the mediating role of risk appraisal for a series of negative life events including a variety of health problems. They examined all four relationships and expected a positive relationship between previous health behaviour and future behaviour, and an effect of past behaviour on risk appraisal, which in turn should affect future behaviour. Finally, and most important, risk appraisal should still affect future behaviour after controlling for past behaviour. Perfect mediation results if past behaviour does not affect future behaviour when risk appraisal is controlled for (Barron and Kenny, 1986).

The influence of past behaviour on future behaviour is well established (e.g. Bentler and Speckart, 1979; Sutton, in this volume). Most studies in the area of risk perception focus on the relationship between perceived risk and behaviour but do *not* control for previous behaviour. Weinstein (1984) provided a negative answer to the question whether people acknowledge the effects of their own risk behaviour on their risk status. He concluded that 'people seem able and willing to incorporate knowledge about their family history, personality, ... and physical or physiological attributes into their perceptions of their vulnerability, at least to a limited extent, but they seem much poorer at recognizing the relationships between their own actions and their risk of harm' (p. 447).

Two explanations were offered for the absence of a relationship between behaviour and risk appraisal. The first (motivational) explanation claims that to acknowledge that one's own (controllable) behaviour puts one at risk is to threaten one's self-esteem. The second (more cognitive) explanation states that people are unaware of the links between behaviour and risk. Contrary to Weinstein, however, Whitley and Hern's (1991) results support the expected relationship between past behaviour and risk appraisal. Women who had protected themselves more against pregnancy in the prior six months gave lower likelihood estimates of getting pregnant in the next year. In accordance with these findings and the assumption that people behave rationally when assessing their risk status (i.e. acknowledging behavioural risk factors) Otten and Van der Pligt (1992) expected that risky behaviour in the past leads to higher risk appraisals for future negative events.

The mediation hypothesis also involves the relation between risk appraisal and future (intended) behaviour. As argued before, perceived vulnerability or susceptibility is a common element in models that try to explain (protective) behaviour. In accordance with these models one would expect higher risk appraisals to be related to increased willingness to engage in protective behaviour. The final part of the mediation hypothesis concerns the combined effects of risk appraisal and past behaviour on future behaviour. Otten and Van der Pligt (1992) focused on both past behaviour and behavioural expectations about the future to determine the mediational influence of risk appraisal, and expected risk appraisal to have a significant impact on future behaviour *after* controlling for past behaviour.

Both studies conducted by Otten and Van der Pligt (1992) showed a clear relationship between past behaviour and risk appraisal, and between past behaviour and future behaviour. The results also indicated a clear relationship between risk appraisal and future behaviour, but in the opposite direction — higher perceived risk was associated with increased levels of risk in future behaviour. Most importantly, when future behaviour was predicted from both risk appraisal *and* previous behaviour, the effect of risk appraisal on future behaviour disappeared while past behaviour remained a strong predictor of future behaviour. The findings thus suggest a *modest* role for risk appraisal as a determinant of future behaviour.

Other research in this field tends to focus on the direct link between risk appraisal and behavioural intentions or behaviour *without* controlling for past behavioural practices. Lee (1989), for example, found a direct link between risk appraisals and smoking. Smokers' ratings of the risks of smoking to the average smoker were lower than non smokers' ratings, and smokers' ratings of their own risk were lower still. Joseph et al. (1987) investigated AIDS preventive behaviour in a sample of homosexual men and focused on perceived risk and its behavioural, social, and psychological consequences. Univariate analyses showed that perceived risk was related to several measures of subsequent behavioural risk reduction. The effects disappeared, however, after adjustment for sociodemographic variables, initial behaviour, and other factors including knowledge about AIDS, perceived self-efficacy, barriers to behavioural change, and social norms. Taylor et al. (1992) also failed to find a direct relationship between perceived risk and behaviour. High risk estimates were not associated with decreased risk behaviours in the six months following the risk assessment. Bauman and Siegel (1987) suggest that people at risk who employ defensive denial as a coping strategy and are optimistic about their vulnerability tend to engage in more risky practices and also to focus on irrelevant precautions to enhance their feeling of safety.

The last three studies deal with at-risk samples and provide only a partial answer concerning the relationship between optimism, perceived vulnerability, behavioural intentions and future behaviour. Other research (also focusing on AIDS related risks) reveals a modest role for risk appraisal. For instance, a study by Van der Velde et al. (1991) among visitors to an STD clinic showed that after adjustment for other variables, perceived risk and optimism were *not* related to subsequent behaviour. Research on adolescents' risk appraisals and sexual practices confirms those findings (Richard and Van der Pligt, 1991). Factors such as self-efficacy and anticipated regret were far more important predictors of preventive behaviour. Overall, the predictive power of comparative risk appraisal seems even more modest. Research incorporating both assessment of one's own risks and comparative risk appraisal (i.e. level of optimism) shows that the former is modestly related to behavioural intentions and actual behaviour (see for example Van der Velde et al., 1992; Otten and Van der Pligt, 1992). Comparative risk appraisal does not add much to the prediction of behaviour over and above perceived (absolute) risk. It could be that comparative risk appraisal serves mainly to trigger social comparison processes and is not a prime determinant of preventive health behaviours.

In summary, after adjustment for other variables, perceived risk and optimism do appear to be related to behavioural intentions and actual behaviour, but only marginally after controlling for other behavioural determinants. As argued before, people have considerable difficulties with probability assessments and it could well be that factors such as the severity of the consequences, social norms, self-efficacy and also the anticipation of regret and worry are more immediate determinants of health behaviour. This does *not* imply that perceived risk is unimportant as a predictor of health behaviour. Perceived risk (absolute *and* comparative) seems a *necessary* condition but not a sufficient condition for behavioural change — a view that coincides with Weinstein's (1988) 'precaution adoption process'. Weinstein's model assumes a logical process preceding the adoption of preventive action to reduce the threat of negative outcomes for one's health. First, people have to realize that a specific hazard exists. Second, they have to realize that the hazard is significant and can affect people. Third, they have to realize that they are vulnerable to the hazard. After these necessary requirements, behavioural change will be a function of the perceived severity of the consequences for one's health and the efficacy and costs of preventive behaviour.

Conclusion

Most models of (health) behaviour focus on perceived risk as an important determinant of behaviour. Some divide risk into a probability component and a value component (i.e. the likelihood of specific consequences and the evaluation of these possible consequences), while others assess perceived vulnerability and do not require subjects to make numerical or verbal probability assessments. In this chapter I have focused on the probability component of risk perception. A number of biases affect both absolute and comparative risk appraisal, and can hinder behavioural change. Health education campaigns should address these issues, for perceived vulnerability is a necessary condition for behavioural change.

Present research does not allow firm conclusions to be drawn about the predictive power of perceived risk as a determinant of preventive action. Generally, perceived risk seems necessary for behavioural change, but is not sufficient. When tested in the context of other behavioural determinants, it is a modest predictor of preventive health behaviour. Comparative risk appraisal serves a number of functions but is not a prime determinant of behaviour.

It could well be that the probability component of risk plays only a marginal role and that the severity of the consequences is a more important determinant of health behaviour. In other words, perceived risk (i.e. probability x value) could well be primarily determined by the severity of the possible consequences. This seems to be the case with large scale technological risk (see for example Van der Pligt, 1992). Research in that field suggests that qualitative aspects of the possible consequences are the prime determinant of risk acceptance, but more research is needed to assess the precise role of perceived risk as a necessary factor. The new research should preferably be *prospective*, for too many studies have assessed perceived risk and behavioural intentions at the same time, which makes it difficult to investigate the predictive power of perceived risk. Also, more attention should be paid to the *measurement* of perceived risk. The many different ways in which perceived risk and vulnerability have been measured make it difficult to compare research outcomes. Most models require a *conditional* probability assessment; most research, however, relies on general, unconditional risk appraisals.

When people are confronted with relatively immediate risks that pose a severe threat, motivational factors play a major role. However, motivational factors can result in substantial biases in risk perception, which poses important problems for health education: a direct confrontational approach could have potentially adverse consequences for those who perceive themselves to be at risk. The complex dual aim of health education programmes is to inform and to create and maintain a level of anxiety that is sufficient to motivate risk reducing behaviours, but which at the same time is not too high. For these reasons it is essential that health education programmes also stress *how* to change behaviour and take preventive action.

References

Ajzen, I. (1985), 'From intentions to actions: a theory of planned behaviour', in Kuhl, J. and Beckmann, J. (eds), *Action-Control: From Cognition to Behavior*, Springer, Heidelberg, pp. 11-39.

Ajzen, I. (1991), 'The Theory of Planned Behavior', *Organizational Behavior and Human Decision Processes*, 50, pp. 179-211.

Bakker, A.B., Buunk, A.P. and Siero, F.W. (1994), 'Condom use of heterosexuals: a comparison of the Theory of Planned Behavior, the Health Belief Model, and protection motivation theory', manuscript submitted for publication.

Bandura, A. (1989), 'Perceived self-efficacy in the exercise of control over AIDS-infection', in Blumenthal, S., Echler, A., and Weissman, G. (eds), *Women and AIDS*, American Psychiatric Press, Washington, DC.

Bauman, L.J., and Siegel, K. (1987), 'Risk perception among gay men of the risk of AIDS associated with their sexual behavior', *Journal of Applied Social Psychology*, 17, pp. 329-350.

Baron, R.M., and Kenny, D.A. (1986), 'The moderator-mediator variable distinction in social psychological research: conceptual, strategic and statistical considerations', *Journal of Personality and Social Psychology*, 51, pp. 1173-1182.

Beale, D.A., and Manstead, A.S.R. (1991), 'Predicting mothers' intentions to limit frequency of infants' sugar intake: testing the Theory of Planned Behavior', *Journal of Applied Social Psychology*, 21, pp. 409-431.

Becker, M.H., Haefner, D.P., Kasl, S.V., Kirscht, J.P., Maiman, L.A., and Rosenstock, J.M. (1977), 'Selected psychosocial models and correlates of individual health-related behaviors', *Medical Care*, 15 (Supplement), pp. 27-46.

Bentler, P.M., and Speckart, G. (1979), 'Models of attitude-behavior relations', *Psychological Review*, 86, pp. 452-464.

Cummings, K.M., Jette, A.M., Brock, B.M., and Haefner, D.P. (1979), 'Psychological determinants of immunization behavior in a Swine Influenza campaign', *Medical Care*, 17, pp. 639-649.

De Vries, H. Dijkstra, M., and Kuhlman, P. (1988), 'Self-efficacy: the third factor besides attitude and subjective norm as a predictor of behavioral intentions', *Health Education Research*, 3, pp. 273-282.

Edwards, W. (1954), 'The theory of decision making', *Psychological Bulletin*, 51, pp. 380-417.

Fischhoff, B., Lichtenstein, S., Slovic, P., Derby, S.L., and Keeney, R.L. (1981), *Acceptable Risk*, Cambridge University Press, Cambridge.

Fishbein, M., and Ajzen, I. (1975), *Beliefs, Attitude, Intention, and Behavior: An Introduction to Theory and Research*, Addison-Wesley, Reading, MA.

Fisher, J.D., and Fisher, W.A. (1992), 'Changing AIDS-risk behavior', *Psychological Bulletin*, 111, pp. 455-474.

Gerrard, M., Gibbons, F.X., and Warner, T.D. (1993), 'Perceived vulnerability to AIDS and AIDS preventive behavior: a critical review of the evidence', in Pryor, J. and Reeder, G. (eds), *The Social Psychology of HIV Infection*, Lawrence Erlbaum, Hillsdale, NJ.

Gladis, M.M., Michela, J.L., Walter, H.J., Vaughan, R.D. (1992), 'High school students' perceptions of AIDS risk: realistic appraisal or motivated denial', *Health Psychology*, 11, pp. 307-316.

Harris, D.M., and Guten, S. (1979), 'Health-protective behavior: an exploratory study', *Journal of Health and Social Behavior*, 20, pp. 17-29.

Janis, I.L., and Mann, L. (1977), *Decision Making: A Psychological Analysis of Conflict, Choice, and Commitment*, Free Press, New York.

Janz, N., and Becker, M. (1984), 'The Health Belief Model: a decade later', *Health Education Quarterly*, 11, pp. 1-47.

Joseph, J.G., Montgomery, S.B., Emmons, C.A., Kirscht, J.P., Kessler, R.C., Ostrow, D.G., Wortman, C.B., O'Brien, K., Eller, M., and Eshleman, S. (1987), 'Perceived risk of AIDS: assessing the behavioral and psychological consequences in a cohort of gay men', *Journal of Applied Social Psychology*, 17, pp. 231-250.

Kasl, S.V. (1975), 'Social psychological characteristics associated with behaviors that reduce cardiovascular risk', in Enslow, A.J. and Henderson, J. (eds), *Applying Behavioral Science to Cardiovascular Risk*, American Heart Association, Dallas, pp. 173-180.

Kirscht, J.P. (1983), 'Preventive health behavior: a review of research and issues', *Health Psychology*, 2, pp. 279-301.

Lee, C. (1989), 'Perceptions of immunity to disease in adult smokers', *Journal of Behavioral Medicine*, 12, pp. 267-277.

Leventhal, H., Safer, M.A., and Panagis, D.M. (1983), 'The impact of communications on self-regulation of health beliefs, decisions, and behavior', *Health Education Quarterly*, 10, pp. 3-31.

Madden, T.J., Ellen, P.S., and Ajzen, I. (1992), 'A comparison of the Theory of Planned Behavior and the Theory of Reasoned Action', *Personality and Social Psychology Bulletin*, 18, pp. 3-9.

Montgomery, S.B., Joseph, J.G., Becker, M.H., Ostrow, D.G., Kessler, R.C., and Kirscht, J.P. (1989), 'The Health Belief Model in understanding compliance with preventive recommendations for AIDS: how useful?', *AIDS Education and Prevention*, 1, pp. 303-323.

Otten, W., and Van der Pligt, J. (1992), 'Risk and behavior: the mediating role of risk appraisal', *Acta Psychologica*, 80, pp. 325-346.

Parker, D., Manstead, A.S.R., Stradling, S.G., Reason, J.T., and Baxter, J.S. (1992), 'Intention to commit driving violations: an application of the Theory of Planned Behavior', *Journal of Applied Psychology*, 77, pp. 94-101.

Pechacek, T., and Danaher, B. (1979), 'How and why people quit smoking: a cognitive-behavioral analysis', in Kendall, P. and Hollon, S. (eds), *Cognitive Behavioral Intervention: Theory, Research, and Procedures*, Academic Press, New York, pp. 389-422.

Perloff, L.S., and Farbisz, R. (1985), *Perceptions of Uniqueness and Illusions of Invulnerability to Divorce*, paper presented at the Midwestern Psychological Association Meeting, Chicago.
Richard, R., and Van der Pligt, J. (1991), 'Factors affecting condom use among adolescents', *Journal of Community and Applied Social Psychology*, 1, pp. 105-116.
Rippetoe, P.A., and Rogers, R.W. (1987), 'Effects of components of protection-motivation theory on adaptive and maladaptive coping with a health threat', *Journal of Personality and Social Psychology*, 52, pp. 596-604.
Rogers, R.W. (1975), 'A protection motivation theory of fear appeals and attitude change', *The Journal of Psychology*, 91, pp. 93-114.
Ronis, D.L. (1992), 'Conditional health threats: health beliefs, decisions, and behaviour among adults', *Health Psychology*, 11, pp. 127-134.
Scheier, M.F., and Carver, C.S. (1992), 'Effects of optimism on psychological and physical well-being: theoretical overview and empirical update', *Cognitive Therapy and Research*, 16, pp. 201-228.
Schifter, D.B., and Ajzen, I. (1985), 'Intention, perceived control, and weight loss: an application of the Theory of Planned Behavior', *Journal of Personality and Social Psychology*, 49, pp. 843-851.
Sheppard, B.H., Hartwick, J., and Warshaw, P.R. (1988), 'The Theory of Reasoned Action: a meta-analysis of past research with recommendations for modifications and future research', *Journal of Consumer Research*, 15, pp. 325-343.
Slovic, P., Fischhoff, B., and Lichtenstein, S. (1978), 'Accident probabilities and seat belt usage: a psychological perceptive', *Accident Analysis and Prevention*, 10, pp. 281-285.
Sparks, P., Hedderley, D., and Shepherd, R. (1992), 'An investigation into the relationship between perceived control, attitude variability and the consumption of two common foods', *European Journal of Social Psychology*, 22, pp. 55-71.
Svenson, O. (1981), 'Are we all less risky and more skillful than our fellow drivers?', *Acta Psychologica*, 47, pp. 143-148.
Taylor, S.E., and Brown, J.D. (1988), 'Illusion and well-being: a social-psychological perspective on mental health', *Psychological Bulletin*, 103, pp. 193-210.
Taylor, S.E., Kemeny, M.E., Aspinwall, L.G., Schneider, S.G., Rodriguez, R., and Herbert, M. (1992), 'Optimism, Coping, Psychological Distress, and High-Risk Sexual Behavior among Men at Risk for AIDS', *Journal of Personality and Social Psychology*, 63, pp. 460-473.
Tversky, A., and Kahneman, D. (1974), 'Judgment under uncertainty: heuristics and biases', *Science*, 185, pp. 1127-31.

Van der Pligt, J. (1992), *Nuclear Energy and the Public*, Blackwell, Oxford.
Van der Pligt, J., and Eiser, J.R. (1984), 'Dimensional salience, judgment and attitudes', in Eiser, J.R. (ed.), *Attitudinal Judgment*, Springer Verlag, New York.
Van der Pligt, J., Otten, W., Richard, R., and Van der Velde, F. (1993), 'Perceived risk of AIDS: unrealistic optimism and self-protective action', in Pryor, J. and Reeder, G. (eds), *The Social Psychology of HIV Infection*, Lawrence Erlbaum, Hillsdale, NJ.
Van der Velde, F.W., and Van der Pligt, J. (1991), 'AIDS related health behavior: coping, protection motivation and previous behavior', *Behavioral Medicine*, 14, pp. 429-452.
Van der Velde, F.W., Hooijkaas, C., and Van der Pligt, J. (1992), 'Risk perception and behavior: pessimism, realism, and optimism about AIDS-related health behavior', *Psychology and Health*, 6, pp. 23-28.
Weinstein, N.D. (1980), 'Unrealistic optimism about future life events', *Journal of Personality and Social Psychology*, 39, pp. 806-820.
Weinstein, N.D. (1982), 'Unrealistic optimism about susceptibility to health problems', *Journal of Behavioral Medicine*, 5, pp. 441-460.
Weinstein, N.D. (1983), 'Reducing unrealistic optimism about illness susceptibility', *Health Psychology*, 2, pp. 11-20.
Weinstein, N.D. (1984), 'Why it won't happen to me: perceptions of risk factors and susceptibility', *Health Psychology*, 3, pp. 431-457.
Weinstein, N.D. (1988), 'The precaution adoption process', *Health Psychology*, 7, pp. 355-386.
Weinstein, N.D. (1989), 'Effects of personal experience on self-protective behavior', *Psychological Bulletin*, 105, pp. 31-50.
Whitley, B.E. Jnr, and Hern, A.L. (1991), 'Perceptions of vulnerability to pregnancy and the use of effective contraception', *Personality and Social Psychology Bulletin*, 17, pp. 104-110.

8 Unrealistic optimism in health and safety risks

Vera Hoorens

Introduction

The perception of one's vulnerability to health and safety risks is a focal aspect of risk appraisal and is present in most models of health and safety behaviour (e.g. Ajzen, 1991; Janz and Becker, 1984; Weinstein, 1988). One important source of information concerning one's vulnerability derives from social comparison (for a review on social comparison see Wood, 1989). However, self-serving biases distort the outcome of social comparison processes (Hoorens, 1993). One of these biases is of special importance to the perception of health and safety risks, namely, unrealistic optimism (Weinstein, 1980). In the present chapter, the evidence for unrealistic optimism in the domain of health and safety is reviewed. Cognitive and motivational explanations of the phenomenon are evaluated and its consequences are briefly discussed. Finally, guidelines for future research are pointed out.

Unrealistic optimism in the domain of health and safety: an overview of the evidence

One of the first demonstrations of self-serving bias in the estimation of health risks was provided by Larwood (1978) who showed that most people estimate their own risk of getting flu as lower than the average person's risk. However, the term 'unrealistic optimism' was coined by Weinstein (1980). A majority of his subjects estimated their own chances of experiencing a number of positive events higher, and their own chances of experiencing negative events lower, than their peers' chances. As it is impossible that most members of a population will be better off than the other members (except in very skewed distributions), on the group level this perception may be called illusory or unrealistic. Although Perloff (1983, 1987) describes the biased perception of one's own future as 'the illusion of unique invulnerability', the occurrence of the phenomenon for positive as well as for negative events justifies the more general label 'unrealistic optimism'.

A large number of negative events used by Weinstein (1980, experiment 1) were health and safety hazards such as having a heart attack or being involved in a car accident. Except for cancer, all the risks yielded unrealistic optimism. However, as the response alternatives were unevenly distributed below rather than above average, Weinstein's subjects may have displayed an artefactually strong optimism. In a series of subsequent studies, Weinstein (1982, 1983, 1984, 1987) expanded and improved his original research by using a more balanced response scale and by analysing unrealistic optimism for a wider variety of health risks. Asking for students' own risk estimations 'as compared to other Rutgers students of the same sex' on a seven point scale ranging from much below average (–3) to much above average (+3), Weinstein (1982) demonstrated unrealistic optimism for 34 of a series of 45 health problems. For instance, subjects thought they were less vulnerable than others to infectious hepatitis, sunstroke, and multiple sclerosis. No unrealistic optimism was obtained for a non-specified form of cancer and the common cold. While one health problem (ulcers) yielded unrealistic *pessimism*, later research by the same author showed unrealistic optimism for this hazard as well (Weinstein, 1983, 1984, 1987).

Unrealistic optimism has been demonstrated using different measures, in different subject populations, and for a variety of risks. Besides using relative risk estimations, authors have also measured unrealistic optimism as the difference between subjects' absolute risk estimates for themselves and a comparison other. Using this procedure, Dolinski, Gromski and Zawisza (1987), for instance, found unrealistic optimism for prospects such as being robbed, being involved in a train accident, and having a heart attack. In addition, although most studies on unrealistic optimism have been performed among university students, the phenomenon has also been demonstrated in populations less privileged in terms of age, intelligence and social background. For instance, unrealistic optimism concerning one's risk of getting AIDS has been demonstrated in a representative sample of Dutch citizens (Sandfort, 1991) and among heterosexual men and women with unsteady sexual relationships and who visited a clinic for venereal diseases (Van der Velde, Hooijkaas and Van der Pligt, 1991).

Although unrealistic optimism has been demonstrated for a wide variety of health and safety risks, a limited set of risks has received extensive attention. For most of them, the strength of the effect has been remarkably constant over studies. Unrealistic optimism for HIV infection or AIDS has been found in homosexuals, heterosexuals, representative population samples and visitors to clinics for venereal diseases (besides the studies mentioned earlier see also Bauman and Siegel, 1987; Gerrard, Gibbons and Warner, 1991; Hoorens and Buunk, 1991; Joseph et al., 1987; Schneider et al., 1991; however, see Mannetti and Pierro, 1991, for an exception). Similarly, people generally display unrealistic optimism concerning venereal diseases (e.g. Van der Velde et al., 1991; Perloff and Fetzer, 1986; Weinstein, 1980), heart attacks (e.g. Burger and Palmer, 1992; Dolinski et al., 1987; Hoorens and Buunk, 1991; Perloff and Fetzer, 1986; Van der Velde et al., 1991; Weinstein, 1982; but see Weinstein, 1987), drinking problems (e.g. Burger and Palmer, 1992; Hoorens and Buunk, 1991; Perloff and Fetzer, 1986; Weinstein, 1983), being mugged (Burger and Palmer, 1992; Dolinski et al., 1987; Weinstein, 1984 (study 2), 1987; see Weinstein, 1984 (study 1) for an exception) and being involved in a car accident (e.g. DeJoy, 1989, 1992; Finn and Bragg, 1986; Matthews and Moran, 1986; Svenson, Fischhoff and MacGregor, 1985). The evidence is mixed for the risk of *being injured* in a car accident: while some authors find unrealistic optimism (Dolinski et al., 1987; Weinstein, 1984 (study 2), 1987; Zakay, 1983), others do not (Burger and Palmer, 1992; Perloff and Fetzer, 1986; Weinstein, 1983, 1984 (study 1)) or even obtain unrealistic pessimism (Weinstein, 1980). The same holds for hypertension: about as many studies do (Burger and Palmer, 1992; Perloff and Fetzer, 1986; Weinstein, 1984 (study 2)) as do not (Weinstein, 1982, 1983, 1984 (study 1), 1987) find unrealistic optimism.

Thus far, only one health risk has *not* typically yielded unrealistic optimism, namely unspecified cancer (Burger and Palmer, 1992; Dolinski et al., 1987; Hoorens and Buunk, 1991; McCoy, Gibbons, Reis, Gerrard, Luus and Von Wald Sufka, 1992; Weinstein, 1980, 1982, 1983, 1984, 1987; but see Perloff and Fetzer, 1986). This is the more surprising as unrealistic optimism is usually obtained for *specific* forms of cancer such as lung cancer (Van der Velde et al., 1991; Weinstein, 1980, 1982, 1987; Weinstein and Lachendro, 1982; but see Weinstein, 1983) and skin cancer (Weinstein, 1982, 1987), and for cancer related health risks such as having a radon problem in the house (Sandman, Weinstein and Klotz, 1987; Weinstein, Klotz and Sandman, 1988; Weinstein, Sandman and Roberts, 1990).

Cognitive and motivational explanations

Theoretical debates on biases in social comparison have often focused on the question of whether biases are cognitive or motivational in nature. In the present section, both cognitive and motivational explanations will be critically reviewed and an integration of the two approaches will be suggested.

Cognitive hypotheses

Even when people are motivated to get unbiased and complete social comparison information, it may be impossible for them to do so because information is not available and/or because the complex cognitive tasks involved exceed their cognitive skills. Cognitive explanations for unrealistic optimism include the differential availability of and/or selective attention to information, the inadequate use of base rate information, biased perceptions of control, the use of prototypes in social comparison, and the person positivity bias.

Differential availability of and selective attention to information Whereas people are aware of their own actions to avoid health and safety threats, cognitive egocentrism or a lack of information may inhibit an accurate perception of other people's precautions and of their own endangering habits. Therefore when comparing their own risks to 'the average other's', people may compare a rosily perceived self to a hypothetical person who takes not a single precaution and who displays particularly risky behaviours (Weinstein, 1980; Weinstein, Klotz and Sandman, 1988). This biased comparison process may then feed the belief that one's own risks are relatively low.

Weinstein (1980) found that subjects who listed factors that increased or decreased their own chances of experiencing a number of risks and who were then confronted with the lists of five other subjects showed weaker unrealistic optimism concerning those risks than subjects who did not list their own behaviours before giving estimations or who were not confronted with other people's lists. It seems, then, that being confronted with information on other people's precautions and thus implicitly being forced to consider their point of view decreases unrealistic optimism.

Weinstein and Lachendro (1982) tried to separate the effects of differential availability of information about other people's precautions from the effects of cognitive egocentrism or failure to attend to those precautions. In a factorial design, after providing relative risk estimations for a number of health related and non-health related events, subjects either did or did not list their own precautions and were then divided into three groups. In the first group subjects were provided with another subject's list (information-perspective condition); in a second group subjects were asked to take the perspective of another person and to list this person's precautions (perspective condition); and in a third group subjects received no further treatment (control condition). All subjects were then asked to give relative risk estimations for the same events. Whereas the description of their own behaviour did not change subjects' relative estimations, both taking another person's perspective and being provided with information on another person's precautions resulted in a decrease in unrealistic optimism. No significant differences between the information conditions and the perspective conditions were obtained. Weinstein and Lachendro (1982) concluded from the data that, compared to the differential availability of information, cognitive egocentrism was the more important antecedent of unrealistic optimism.

Weinstein (1983) showed that subjects who rated both themselves and the typical same sex person on a predetermined list of relevant risk factors displayed less unrealistic optimism than subjects who did not consider risk factors. In contrast to the earlier findings, however, subjects who rated only their own risk factors showed stronger unrealistic optimism than controls. Gerrard et al. (1991) explained the results by arguing that the cognitive egocentrism (or 'selective focus') hypothesis predicts that people will attend to their self-protective behaviour more carefully than to their self-endangering behaviour. Scrutinizing one's own risk relevant behaviour should thus enhance unrealistic optimism. The suggestion was supported for unwanted pregnancy but not for HIV infection, the latter risk showing the opposite effect. However, most subjects in the study (sexually active women) did not take the single most obvious precaution against HIV (using condoms) so that little room for self-serving bias in information selection was available to them.

If people pay more attention to their self-protective actions than to their risk behaviours, this should be evident in the nature of the behaviours listed. Weinstein (1987) indeed found that protective factors were named more often than endangering factors (see also Weinstein, 1980). This was especially the case for personal actions and psychological attributes, but less so for hereditary and environmental factors. In addition, subjects ascribed more risk decreasing behaviours and fewer risk increasing behaviours to themselves than to the typical same sex other.

Two types of indirect evidence further support the cognitive egocentrism hypothesis. First, according to DeJoy (1989), the hypothesis is contradicted by the finding that increasing experience within a risk domain is associated with increasing unrealistic optimism (e.g. experienced drivers show stronger unrealistic optimism concerning traffic accidents than less experienced drivers). However, it seems more reasonable to assume that the effect of differential attention to self-protective factors should accumulate with experience. From this point of view, DeJoy's findings (1989, 1992, Svenson et al., 1985, study 2; see, however, Svenson et al., 1985, study 1) support rather than undermine the cognitive egocentrism hypothesis. Moreover, both in the domain of health and safety and in other domains people show unrealistic optimism when the comparison other is a vague instance such as 'the average other' or 'most others', but they do not show it, or show it to a reduced degree, when the other is a familiar person such as their best same sex friend or a sibling (Hoorens and Buunk, 1991; Perloff and Fetzer, 1986). Such results may be interpreted in terms of the greater interest in and knowledge of significant others' self-protective behaviour than 'the average other's'.

The pattern that emerges from the literature review so far is that the information-attention hypothesis has taken various specific forms and that the differences between them have often not been made explicit. On the one hand, it is not always clear whether cognitive egocentrism or the objective availability of information is considered the essential factor. On the other hand, while researchers have sometimes focused on the differential treatment of information concerning one's own risk *reducing* versus risk *increasing* characteristics and behaviours, at other times they have focused on the differential treatment of one's own versus other people's risk reducing attributes. At yet other times they have focused on self-other differences in the relative attendance to risk reducing versus risk increasing attributes.

While 'informational/attentional' explanations of unrealistic optimism have received extensive support, they cannot *completely* explain unrealistic optimism. Indeed, the phenomenon still occurs — albeit to a reduced degree — when subjects are confronted with salient information on other people's risk status. Moreover, even when cognitive egocentrism and the availability of information are clearly distinguished, the evidence is inconclusive as to which factor is the more important in causing unrealistic optimism. Whereas Weinstein and Lachendro (1982) argue in favour of selective focus or cognitive egocentrism, the finding that supplying information about other people did not produce a greater decrease in unrealistic optimism than merely asking people to take another person's perspective may be due to the potential non-additivity of the effects.

Inadequate use of base rate information People may believe that if the a priori probability of undesirable experiences is very small, the probability that *they* will suffer the risk is especially low (Weinstein, 1980). In other words, they may ignore the fact that small probabilities apply to anyone and not particularly to themselves. Stronger unrealistic optimism effects have indeed been obtained for rare health risks than for more common ones (Weinstein, 1982, 1987). However, a closer look at the data reveals that the empirical evidence is rather weak. In Weinstein's (1982, 1987) studies, for example, probability ratings were correlated with other risk dimensions such as ratings of seriousness and personal experience. Multiple regression analyses yielded no independent contribution of probability ratings. Furthermore, neither DeJoy (1989) nor Weinstein (1980) found a relationship between the probability of risks and unrealistic optimism. Taken together, the findings offer no compelling evidence that population probabilities influence unrealistic optimism.

People may go beyond population probabilities as a base rate for estimating their personal risks, and may use their own and their close friends' and relatives' previous experiences. People who have not been confronted with a health or safety risk may infer that their future risks are relatively low as well. As most health and safety risks used in unrealistic optimism research are rather uncommon for the populations under study, it is likely that most subjects have not experienced them already and hence underestimate their own vulnerability for the future.

In line with this view, subjects who report having been victims of the risk or knowing friends or relatives who have been victims show less unrealistic optimism than others (Van der Pligt, 1991; Van der Velde et al., 1991; Weinstein, 1980, 1982, 1987). Illnesses assumed to develop early in life also yield greater unrealistic optimism in non-victims than do illnesses with a later onset (Weinstein, 1987). Furthermore, subjects who show or who have shown extensive risk-related behaviour without being seriously harmed display relatively strong unrealistic optimism. For instance, unrealistic optimism concerning one's chances of being involved in car accidents increases with increasing driving experience. However, the relationship may be due to a realistic perception by more experienced drivers of their greater driving skills. The latter objection does not apply to studies showing greater unrealistic optimism about smoking related health problems in smokers than in ex-smokers or non smokers (McCoy et al., 1992; see, however, Lee, 1989).

Apparently, the effect of previous experience is highly risk specific. Shortly after the Chernobyl disaster Polish subjects showed unrealistic optimism for non-radiation related health and safety risks but unrealistic pessimism concerning radiation related health problems (Dolinski et al., 1987). In addition, the effects appear to dissipate over time. Although Californian subjects did not show unrealistic optimism when estimating their risk of 'being seriously hurt in a natural disaster' shortly after an earthquake, they did a few months later (Burger and Palmer, 1992). Similarly, unrealistic optimism concerning one's chances of getting flu or other health problems was found to be positively correlated with the length of time since one's most recent health problem (Larwood, 1978). Taken together, these and the earlier findings we have discussed thus offer good support for the hypothesis that an inadequate use of base rate information derived from one's own previous experience is an important determinant of risk specific unrealistic optimism.

Biased perception of control If diseases, crimes and accidents are easily avoidable, people may take the necessary precautions and hence reduce their risks. Unrealistic optimism may emerge if people overestimate the degree to which they can control the risks relative to other people, if they overlook the action others take to exert their control, and/or if they believe that they possess the necessary skills to a larger degree than others.

Two lines of evidence support the controllability view. First, greater unrealistic optimism has been obtained for subjectively controllable risks than for uncontrollable hazards (DeJoy, 1989; Van der Pligt, 1991; Van der Velde et al., 1991; Weinstein, 1980, 1982, 1987; Zakay, 1984). Second, subjects with an internal locus of control or with a strong desire for control show stronger personal optimism than people with an external locus of control (Drake, 1987; Hoorens and Buunk, 1991).

What is the mechanism by which locus of control is linked to unrealistic optimism? One possibility is that people relatively overestimate their own personal control. In a non-health and safety related context, Brinthaupt, Picone and Moreland (1990) found that students perceived the benefits they expected to gain from membership of a student organization as more controllable than those to be gained by other students. Similarly, Martin, Abramson and Alloy (1984) found that male subjects overestimated the degree to which they could control a truly non-contingent experimental outcome, but correctly judged that a confederate exerted little control. However, even in the absence of any control-related self-other difference, differential attention to one's own and other people's precautions may lead to control dependent unrealistic optimism.

There is also considerable evidence that people overestimate their own abilities and desirable characteristics in comparison with other people's abilities and characteristics (e.g. Alicke, 1985; Marks, 1984). To the extent that such attributes are necessary or useful for taking the relevant precautions, one's own future should look brighter than other people's futures. For instance, people typically believe they are better and safer drivers than others (e.g. DeJoy, 1989, 1992; Delhomme, 1991; Goszczynska and Roslan, 1989; Matthews and Moran, 1986), making a subjective invulnerability to traffic accidents readily understandable. In one of their studies, Svenson et al. (1985) found that subjects who believed themselves to be particularly safe and skilled drivers also strongly believed that they were relatively invulnerable to road accidents (see also DeJoy, 1989). Further underlining the close relationship between illusory superiority and unrealistic optimism, the two phenomena covary with identical factors. For instance, increased driving experience is associated with perceived superiority concerning one's driving skills (Groeger and Brown, 1989) as well as with personal optimism concerning road accidents. Hoorens and Buunk (1992a; see also Hoorens, 1993, 1994) even showed that personal optimism and perceived superiority are still closely related when the abilities and traits under study are not specifically associated with the prospects presented to subjects.

Prototypes in social comparison People may believe themselves to be relatively invulnerable because they compare themselves to a prototypical victim rather than to 'the average person' or 'others in general' (Weinstein, 1980; DeJoy, 1989). It is assumed in this view that the cognitive representation of a given health or safety hazard includes an image of the prototypical risk person and that this image is activated whenever people are confronted with the hazard under study. When people try to imagine the 'average other', their mental image is replaced or at least distorted by the relevant victim prototype so that the comparison other is a high risk person, leading to a relative underestimation of one's own risks.

Indirect evidence for the prototype view may be derived from findings that show little or no unrealistic optimism when instructions prevent subjects using a prototypical comparison other — when, for example, they are instructed to compare themselves to a well known other (see above). However, such a pattern of results is also predicted by hypotheses that focus on the differential availability of or attention to self- and other-related information.

Also in line with the prototype hypothesis, unrealistic optimism is associated with a greater rated imaginability of the type of person who would be confronted with the hazard under study (DeJoy, 1989; Weinstein, 1980; see, however, Weinstein, 1982). However, one important problem with these studies is that subjects were asked to rate the degree to which they could imagine either a high risk person or the threat itself. There is no guarantee that subjects' ratings are an accurate reflection of their real capacity to imagine the relevant persons or events. It is possible that unrealistic optimism is associated with a subjective *feeling* of being able to imagine a typical victim but not with his or her 'real' imaginability.

Person positivity bias People often value the members of a group more positively than the group as a whole (Sears, 1983). In many studies on unrealistic optimism, subjects compare their future to the future of a comparison other implicitly or explicitly referring to a group such as 'the average other' (Perloff, 1987) or 'other same sex students of the same university' (e.g. Weinstein, 1980). Unrealistic optimism may thus be a side effect of the 'person positivity bias'.

The person positivity explanation seems at first sight to be supported by the finding that unrealistic optimism is reduced or eliminated when the comparison other is one's best friend or a sibling. However, significant others are also better known and better liked than 'the average other'. To try to disentangle the effects, Hoorens and Buunk (1991) asked subjects to compare their own (health) risks to those of an average peer, a randomly chosen peer, and their best friend. Unrealistic optimism was obtained in both the 'random other' and the 'average other' conditions but not in the 'best friend' condition. The results thus contradicted the person positivity explanation.

Motivational hypotheses

The motivational approach to self related biases rests on the assumption that the biases are deliberate distortions of a potentially known reality. The distortions are assumed to be instrumental in obtaining desirable outcomes or avoiding undesirable outcomes. Three motives may be especially relevant in the domain of self related biases, namely self-enhancement, striving for reassurance, and self-presentation. Each will be addressed in the present section.

Self-enhancement Unrealistic optimism may derive from a desire to boost one's apparent competence and self-worth by perceiving oneself as better than others. Indeed, one way of being better is heading for a better future with more desirable experiences and fewer or less serious problems (Weinstein, 1989). If the hypothesis is correct, people who strongly believe that they are better than others should also show relatively strong personal optimism. A link between perceived superiority and personal optimism has indeed been demonstrated. In addition, unrealistic optimism should be stronger for controllable risks than for uncontrollable risks, since failing to avoid a controllable risk is more threatening to one's self-esteem than failing to avoid an uncontrollable risk. As discussed above, controllable risks indeed elicit stronger unrealistic optimism than do uncontrollable risks. Furthermore, the self-enhancement hypothesis is supported by the finding that individual differences in personal optimism are positively related to self-esteem (Hoorens, 1994).

Self-reassurance People may relatively underestimate their own risk of experiencing undesirable events in order to reduce their fear and protect their ego against the threats associated with facing unwanted outcomes. In line with this hypothesis, a number of studies have yielded greater unrealistic optimism for subjectively serious problems than for less serious problems (Dewberry, Ing, James, Nixon, and Richardson, 1990; Perloff, 1987; Weinstein, 1982). However, other studies have yielded no relationship between rated seriousness and personal optimism (DeJoy, 1989; Van der Pligt, 1991; Van der Velde et al., 1991; Weinstein, 1980, 1987). Since the results are inconsistent, and since the risks used in the respective studies range from a variety of health risks (e.g. Weinstein, 1982) to a heterogeneous list of health and non-health risks (e.g. Weinstein, 1980) to a small number of very similar hazards (e.g. DeJoy, 1989; Van der Velde et al., 1991), it is extremely difficult to draw any conclusion.

One line of evidence seems to contradict the relationship between seriousness and optimism. People with a low level of state anxiety generally display a stronger bias than anxious people (e.g. Dewberry and Richardson, 1990; Hoorens and Buunk, 1991). Similarly, Weinstein (1982, 1983; see also DeJoy, 1989) found an inverse relationship between unrealistic optimism associated with health and safety risks and the degree to which subjects reported worrying about the risks (but see Svenson et al., 1985). However, it should be remembered that seriousness ratings are risk ratings, while ratings of worry and anxiety are essentially self-ratings. It is therefore possible that ratings of 'worrying' tap an affective consequence of risk perception and unrealistic optimism, while ratings of 'seriousness' tap one of its determinants.

Probably the most problematic finding for the self-reassurance hypothesis is the observation that unrealistic optimism is greater for controllable than for uncontrollable risks and that people with an internal locus of control show stronger optimism than people with an external locus of control. In the face of unavoidable risks, as noted by DeJoy (1989), denial may be the only way to cope. If unrealistic optimism serves the goal of ego defence, it should be stronger for uncontrollable hazards and for people with an external rather than an internal locus of control.

Overall, there is no consistent evidence for the self-reassurance hypothesis, in that serious threats do not always elicit especially strong unrealistic optimism. Moreover, the direct relationship between perceived control and unrealistic optimism is at odds with predictions derived from the hypothesis.

Self-presentation People may not believe that their future will be rosier than other people's futures, but they may present themselves as uniquely invulnerable in order to display a socially desirable positive outlook on life. Hoorens and Buunk (1992b) tested such a hypothesis by comparing risk estimations given in private and anonymous circumstances with estimations that were believed to be public and identifiable. The two conditions produced similar levels of unrealistic optimism, and there was no support for the self-presentation hypothesis. However, stable individual differences in self-presentational tendencies may be more important determinants of unrealistic optimism than temporary situational variations. Hoorens (1994) therefore reassessed the relationship between self-presentation and superiority biases by relating individual differences in self-deception and impression management to unrealistic optimism. Students who were relatively strongly motivated to present a favourable image to others were more likely to report that they would not experience negative events (including a number of health and safety hazards) than the average student, while self-deception was unrelated to unrealistic optimism about negative events. It seems, then, that individual differences in impression management are associated with individual differences in personal optimism.

Summary and conclusion

Cognitive and motivational explanations of unrealistic optimism have been evaluated. Consistent support has been found for hypotheses focusing on the differential attention to and availability of information, previous experience, perceptions of control, and self-enhancement. Weaker evidence has been found for the role of person prototypes and self-presentation. The person positivity explanation and the self-reassurance view have generally been contradicted.

How can our conclusions be integrated? As noted by Hoorens (1993), motivational hypotheses may describe the 'why' of self-serving biases, while cognitive views describe the 'how' of their emergence. In the case of unrealistic optimism, it seems likely that people strive for a favourable view of their future because they are motivated to develop and maintain a favourable self-image. To construct a favourable yet believable self-image, they attend differentially to self- and other-related information and carefully select 'useful' comparison persons. However, as they do sometimes experience the risk, the confrontation with reality results in a temporary, risk specific, reduction of unrealistic optimism.

Consequences and implications of unrealistic optimism

Taylor and Brown (1988) suggested that positive self-illusions are generally adaptive in that they promote several aspects of mental health. Unrealistic optimism, they argued, contributes to people's happiness, to their ability to care for others, and to their capacity for productive and creative work. In contrast to this rosy view, most researchers on unrealistic optimism in the domain of health and safety predict that the phenomenon will prevent people taking appropriate precautions and appreciating the implications of mass media health education programs for their own lives (e.g. Gerrard et al., 1991). For instance, Slovic, Fischhoff and Lichtenstein (1978) suggest that people may be unwilling to use safety belts because they believe that car accidents will not happen to them. In this section, the behavioural and affective consequences of unrealistic optimism will be reviewed and the implications for health education will be discussed.

Unrealistic optimism, well-being and risk relevant behaviour

High levels of personal optimism are typically associated with low levels of anxiety and worry and high levels of self-esteem. In addition to the evidence cited above, Joseph et al. (1987) found that male homosexuals who thought they were relatively vulnerable to AIDS showed more indications of psychosocial distress six months later than more optimistic students. Schneider et al. (1991) found that in HIV positive (but not in HIV negative) gay men, suicide intent was positively related to subjective relative vulnerability to developing full blown AIDS. Unrealistic optimism, it seems, has a benign effect on people's general well-being and specific worries, especially in threatening situations.

Turning to perceived relative invulnerability and risk relevant behaviour, a number of authors have found positive correlations between personal optimism, endangering behaviour, and neglect of precaution. After the Chernobyl disaster, for example, Polish subjects who perceived themselves as relatively invulnerable to radiation-caused illness were less likely to report taking precautions than subjects who thought they were at no less risk than others (Dolinski et al., 1987). Moreover, Larwood (1978) showed that subjects who were strongly optimistic concerning their chances of getting flu were less willing to get inoculated. Similarly, Weinstein (1982, 1983) found that illnesses that elicited stronger unrealistic optimism were associated with less worry and hence with less interest in taking precautions than illnesses that elicited weaker unrealistic optimism.

Other authors have found no relationship between personal optimism and willingness to take precautions. For instance, no relationship has been found between perceived vulnerability to traffic accidents and willingness to buy insurance (Robertson, 1977) or to use seat belts (Svenson et al., 1985, study 2). A number of studies have even shown that drivers who describe themselves as *less* vulnerable to traffic accidents than average report using their seat belts *more* often than less optimistic drivers, thus yielding inverse relationships between personal optimism, endangering behaviour, and precaution (Svenson et al., 1985, study 1; Weinstein, Grubb and Vautier, 1986). Similarly, Hoorens and Buunk (1991) obtained a positive relationship between self-descriptions of health behaviour (e.g. having regular hours of sleep) and personal optimism.

All the studies described above used self-descriptions and were essentially retrospective or cross-sectional in nature. Using actual behaviour as a dependent variable, Weinstein et al. (1990) found that people who thought the geological radon level in their own house was relatively low were less likely to order a radon test kit than people who thought the level might be relatively high. Again, in a six month longitudinal study among male homosexuals, Joseph et al. (1987) examined the relationship between self-descriptions of sexual behaviour and absolute and relative estimations of vulnerability to HIV infection. After factors such as sociodemographic variables and initial behaviour had been controlled, risk perceptions failed to predict changes in sexual behaviour. Similar results were obtained by Aspinwall, Kemeny, Taylor, Schneider and Dudley (1991). However, the participants in both studies knew their antibody status and belonged to a relatively homogeneous risk group, so that little room may have been left for the detection of a significant perception-behaviour relationship. In addition, absolute and relative risk estimations were combined into a single score so that the specific contribution of perceived self-other differences to the relationships obtained is impossible to determine. Finally, Van der Velde et al. (1991) found that people who believed themselves to be less at risk than their peers from HIV reported a greater intention to take precautions against HIV infection than people who believed that they were more or equally at risk. When asked four months later, optimists indeed reported having taken the least behavioural risk. Again, however, the best predictor of subsequent behaviour was previous behaviour.

It should be clear from the above review that the evidence on the relationship between unrealistic optimism and risk relevant behaviour is highly inconsistent. In the domain of AIDS and HIV, Gerrard, Gibbons, Warner and Smith (1992) interpreted the inconsistencies in terms of the methodological problems associated with retrospective and cross-sectional designs (e.g. self-presentational and rationalization tendencies or memory distortions). One especially intriguing paradox in cross-sectional and retrospective studies is worth considering in more detail. If, indeed, optimism and desirable risk relevant behaviour are positively related, then it is as reasonable to predict that optimists will show *fewer* desirable risk relevant behaviours because they see themselves as invulnerable, as it is to predict that they will show *more* desirable risk relevant behaviours because an originally high vulnerability has led them to adopt a safe and healthy lifestyle, on which perceptions of relative invulnerability may be based (Svenson et al., 1985; Gerrard et al., 1992). It is of paramount importance to apply longitudinal or experimental designs in the causal analysis of unrealistic optimism. However, the limitations of the prospective studies mentioned above (see also Gerrard et al., 1992) and the limited range of risks to which they have been applied render it highly premature to conclude from them that unrealistic optimism has little effect on risk relevant behaviour.

Unrealistic optimism and the effectiveness of mass media campaigns

It has often been suggested that unrealistic optimism reduces the effectiveness of campaigns designed to promote healthy or safe lifestyles (e.g. Svenson, 1981; Weinstein et al., 1988). If people perceive themselves as relatively invulnerable, mass media messages may be perceived as meant only for others. In line with this reasoning, Tyler and Cook (1984) found that media campaigns influence subjects' risk estimations for the general population but not for themselves. However, the exact role of unrealistic optimism in the effectiveness of mass media health and safety campaigns has yet to be studied in detail. The same holds for the potential effect of unrealistic optimism on more specific problems such as patient delay or the time interval between the experience of symptoms and obtaining help. It has been suggested indeed that subjectively invulnerable people take longer to interpret ambiguous unusual sensations as symptoms of serious medical problems, and hence let more time elapse before seeking crucial medical help (Jones, 1990).

In order to decrease the potentially adverse influence of unrealistic optimism on the effectiveness of health and safety education, the relevant information should be presented in such a way that unrealistic optimism has relatively little chance to interfere. For instance, many media campaigns confront people with exemplary peers who are confronted with a given hazard. It is then hoped that they will compare themselves to the exemplar and draw the relevant conclusions for their own lives. However, people show less unrealistic optimism when they consider their own risks before considering someone else's risks (Dolinski et al., 1987; Hoorens and Buunk, 1991; see, however, Perloff and Fetzer, 1986, study 1) or when they compare others to themselves rather than themselves to others

(Hoorens, 1994). The aversive effects of unrealistic optimism may therefore be reduced by encouraging people to consider their own behaviour and their own vulnerability before confronting them with exemplary peers.

Summary and conclusion

A quite consistent body of evidence exists on the positive relationship between psychosocial well-being and unrealistic optimism. In contrast, the effects of unrealistic optimism in the domain of health and safety education have received little attention. Systematic research on the relationship is a matter of high priority. The same, though for different reasons, holds for the relationship between health and safety behaviour and unrealistic optimism. Indeed, inconsistent results and methodological ambiguities hinder any firm conclusion on the optimism-behaviour relationship.

Taken as a whole, should unrealistic optimism be regarded as beneficial or as harmful? The answer depends in part on the answers to the open questions outlined above. In the meantime, several views have been developed on the desirability of biases in social comparison. While Taylor and Brown (1988) defend their positive consequences, Janoff-Bulman (1989) states that illusions are adaptive as long as they operate at the level of people's highest order assumptions about the world and themselves (e.g. I have relatively little to fear about my health). As soon as more specific and lower order assumptions are distorted (e.g. even if I smoke two packets of cigarettes a day I will not get lung cancer), they may become maladaptive. According to Baumeister (1989), the adaptiveness of positive self-illusions such as unrealistic optimism depends on their extremity. In his view there exists an optimal margin of illusion at which the adaptive consequences are maximal and the maladaptive effects are relatively small. In other words, people who believe they are slightly less vulnerable than others may enjoy an enhanced well-being without displaying endangering behaviours. If they believe they are *much* less vulnerable, however, they may display self-destructive behaviours or expose themselves to worse stress if and when they do experience the risks.

Unrealistic optimism: guidelines for future research

Some important methodological considerations may be derived from the present review. They concern the criteria for terming a given risk estimation 'unrealistic', the interpretation of correlations between optimism and personality or situational factors, and the use of self-report measures in the causal analysis of the phenomenon.

As noted earlier, the term 'unrealistic optimism' implies the unavoidable inaccuracy, on a group level, of people's perceptions of their relative invulnerability. However, in the absence of objective risk indicators it is impossible to tell whether a given individual risk estimate should be called unrealistic. Research on individual differences in relative risk perceptions cannot unequivocally be interpreted in terms of *unrealistic* optimism. At most, individual differences may reflect *personal* optimism that may be, but is not necessarily, unrealistic. Future research should therefore be planned strategically to allow for unequivocal conclusions to be drawn about the relationship between unrealistic optimism and its assumed causes and consequences — by examining optimism about different types of risk rather than individual differences in optimism overall, or by comparing meaningful populations that differ on 'within group' unrealistic optimism.

Even if individual and between-risk differences in relative risk estimations could be interpreted unequivocally, most evidence on the relationship between unrealistic optimism and personality or risk variables is correlational in nature. Firm conclusions as to whether a given correlate should be considered a cause or an effect are therefore impossible. Research on unrealistic optimism would profit greatly from a more experimental orientation in which the phenomenon and its assumed antecedents were manipulated explicitly. Whenever practical or ethical reasons inhibit such a manipulation, longitudinal studies offer a more effective alternative than a cross-sectional or retrospective approach.

Another problem in research on unrealistic optimism has to do with the measurement of its assumed causes and consequences. Most researchers have used self-report measures of constructs such as risk relevant behaviour, interest in taking precautions, and availability of person prototypes. However, as noted already, there is no guarantee that self-descriptions are accurate measures of the relevant behavioural or cognitive variables. In order to obtain unequivocal results on the causal structure of unrealistic optimism, more construct-valid measures of both its causes and its consequences are highly desirable.

Conclusion

Evidence for unrealistic optimism in the domain of health and safety has been reviewed. It has been suggested that the phenomenon may best be explained by means of an integration of cognitive and motivational factors. More specifically, striving for a favourable self-image has been put forward as the motivational force behind people's differential attention to self- and other-related information and their careful selection of 'useful' comparison persons. One consequence of the resulting unrealistic optimism is an enhanced psychosocial well-being; the consequences for risk relevant behaviour and for mass media health and safety promotion remain unclear.

References

Ajzen, I. (1991), 'The Theory of Planned Behaviour', *Organizational Behaviour and Human Decision Processes*, 50, pp. 179-211.

Alicke, M.D. (1985), 'Global self-evaluation as determined by the desirability and controllability of trait adjectives', *Journal of Personality and Social Psychology*, 49, pp. 1621-1630.

Aspinwall, L.G., Kemeny, M.E., Taylor, S.E. and Schneider, S.G. (1991), 'Psychosocal predictors of gay men's AIDS risk-reduction behavior', *Health Psychology*, 10, pp. 432-444.

Bauman, L.J. and Siegel, K. (1987), 'Misperception among gay men of the risk for AIDS associated with their sexual behavior', *Journal of Applied Social Psychology*, 17, pp. 329-350.

Baumeister, R.F. (1989), 'The optimal margin of illusion', *Journal of Social and Clinical Psychology*, 8, pp. 176-189.

Brinthaupt, T.M., Picone, J.J. and Moreland, R.L. (1990), *Self-enhancement, Information Sources, and the Optimism of Prospective Group Members*, paper presented at the Annual Meeting of the Midwestern Psychological Association, Chicago, May 1990.

Burger, J.M. and Palmer, M.L. (1992), 'Changes in and generalization of unrealistic optimism following experiences with stressful events: reactions to the 1989 California eartquake', *Personality and Social Psychology Bulletin*, 18, pp. 39-43.

DeJoy, D.M. (1989), 'The optimism bias and traffic accident risk perception', *Accident Analysis and Prevention*, 21, pp. 333-340.

DeJoy, D.M. (1992), 'An examination of gender differences in traffic accident risk perception', *Accident Analysis and Prevention*, 24, pp. 237-246.

Delhomme, P. (1991), 'Comparing one's driving with others's: assessment of abilities and frequency of offences. Evidence for a superior conformity of self-bias?', *Accident Analysis and Prevention*, 23, pp. 493-508.

Dewberry, C., Ing, M., James, S., Nixon, M. and Richardson, S. (1990), 'Anxiety and unrealistic optimism', *Journal of Social Psychology*, 130, pp. 151-156.

Dewberry, C. and Richardson, S. (1990), 'Effect of anxiety on optimism', *Journal of Social Psychology*, 130, pp. 731-738.

Dolinski, D., Gromski, W. and Zawisza, E. (1987), 'Unrealistic pessimism', *Journal of Social Psychology*, 127, pp. 511-516.

Drake, R.A. (1987), 'Conceptions of own versus others' outcomes: manipulation by monaural attentional orientation', *European Journal of Social Psychology*, 17, pp. 373-375.

Finn, B. and Bragg, W.E. (1986), 'Perception of the risk of an accident by younger and older drivers', *Accident Analysis and Prevention*, 18, pp. 289-298.

Gerrard, M., Gibbons, F.X. and Warner, T.D. (1991), 'Effects of reviewing risk-relevant behavior on perceived vulnerability', *Health Psychology*, 10, pp. 173-179.

Gerrard, M., Gibbons, F.X., Warner, T.D. and Smith, G.E. (1992), 'Perceived vulnerability to HIV infection and AIDS preventive behavior: a critical review of the evidence', in Pryor, J.B. and Reeder, G. (eds), *The Social Psychology of HIV Infection*, Lawrence Erlbaum, Hillsdale, NJ.

Goszczynska, M. and Roslan, A. (1989), 'Self-evaluation of drivers' skill: a cross-cultural comparison', *Accident Analysis and Prevention*, 21, pp. 217-224.

Groeger, J.A. and Brown, I.D. (1989), 'Assessing one's own and others' driving ability: influences of sex, age, and experience', *Accident Analysis and Prevention*, 21, pp. 155-168.

Hoorens, V. (1993), 'Self-enhancement and superiority biases in social comparison', in Stroebe, W. and Hewstone, M. (eds), *European Review of Social Psychology*, Vol. 4, Wiley, Chichester, pp. 113-139.

Hoorens, V. (1994), 'Superiority biases, self-presentation and the self-other asymmetry in social comparison', *Journal of Personality* (in press).

Hoorens, V. and Buunk, A.P. (1991), *Social Comparison of Health Risks*, paper presented at the European Association of Experimental Social Psychology Small Group Meeting: Social Psychological Models in Health and Safety Research, University of Kent at Canterbury, September 1991.

Hoorens, V. and Buunk, A.P. (1992a), 'Zelfdienende vertekeningen in sociale vergelijking: illusoire superioriteit en onrealistisch optimisme', *Psychologica Belgica*, 32, pp. 169-194.

Hoorens, V. and Buunk, A.P. (1992b), 'Onrealistisch optimisme met betrekking tot positieve en negatieve toekomstverwachtingen: de rol van sociale wenselijkheid en de vergelijkingsander', in Ellemers, N., Van der Kloot, W., Poppe, T. and Van der Pligt, T. (eds), *Fundamentele Sociale Psychologie*, Vol. 6, Tilburg University Press, Tilburg, pp. 145-156.

Janoff-Bulman, R. (1989), 'The benefits of illusions, the threat of disillusionment, and the limitations of inaccuracy', *Journal of Social and Clinical Psychology*, 8, pp. 130-157.

Janz, J.K. and Becker, M.H. (1984), 'The Health Belief Model: a decade later', *Health Education Quarterly*, 11, pp. 1-47.

Jones, R.A. (1990), 'Expectations and delay in seeking medical care', *Journal of Social Issues*, 46, pp. 81-95.

Joseph, J.G., Montgomery, S.B., Emmons, C.-A., Kirscht, J.P., Kessler, R.C., Ostrow, D.G., Wortman, C.B., O'Brien, K., Eller, M. and Eshleman, S. (1987), 'Perceived risk of AIDS: assessing the behavioral and psychosocial consequences in a cohort of gay men', *Journal of Applied Social Psychology*, 17, pp. 231-250.

Larwood, L. (1978), 'Swine Flu: a field study of self-serving bias', *Journal of Applied Social Psychology*, 8, pp. 283-289.

Lee, C. (1989), 'Perceptions of immunity to disease in adult smokers', *Journal of Behavioral Medicine*, 12, pp. 267-277.

Mannetti, L. and Pierro, A. (1991), 'Health care workers' reactions to AIDS victims: perception of risk and attribution of responsibility', *Journal of Community and Applied Social Psychology*, 1, pp. 133-142.

Marks, G. (1984), 'Thinking one's abilities are unique and one's opinions are common', *Personality and Social Psychology Bulletin*, 10, pp. 203-208.

Martin, D.J., Abramson, L.Y. and Alloy, L.B. (1984), 'The illusion of control for self and others in depressed and nondepressed college students', *Journal of Personality and Social Psychology*, 46, pp. 125-136.

Matthews, M.L. and Moran, A.R. (1986), 'Age differences in male drivers' perception of accident risk: the role of perceived driving ability', *Accident Analysis and Prevention*, 18, pp. 205-208.

McCoy, S.B., Gibbons, F.X., Reis, T.J., Gerrard, M., Luus, C.A.E. and Von Wald Sufka, A. (1992), 'Perceptions of smoking risk as a function of smoking status', *Journal of Behavioral Medicine*, 15, pp. 469-488.

Perloff, L.S. (1983), 'Perceptions of vulnerability to victimization', *Journal of Social Issues*, 39, pp. 41-61.

Perloff, L.S. (1987), 'Social comparison and illusions of invulnerability to negative life events', in Snyder, C.R. and Ford, C. (eds), *Coping with Negative Life Events: Clinical and Psychological Perspectives*, New York, Plenum Press.

Perloff, L.S. and Fetzer, B.K. (1986), 'Self-other judgments and perceived vulnerability to victimization', *Journal of Personality and Social Psychology*, 50, pp. 502-510.

Robertson, L.S. (1977), 'Car crashes: perceived vulnerability and willingness to pay for crash protection', *Journal of Community Health*, 3, pp. 136-141.

Sandfort, T. (1991), 'Hoe onveilig vrijt Nederland?', in Van Zessen, G. and Sandfort, T. (eds), *Seksualiteit in Nederland. Seksueel gedrag, risico en preventie van AIDS*, Swets and Zeitlinger, Amsterdam.

Sandman, P.M., Weinstein, N.D. and Klotz, M.L. (1987), 'Public response to the risk from geological radon', *Journal of Communication*, 37, pp. 93-108.

Schneider, S.G., Taylor, S.E., Hammen, C., Kemeny, M. E. and Dudley, J. (1991), 'Factors influencing suicide intent in gay and bisexual suicide ideators: differing models for men with and without human immunodeficiency virus', *Journal of Personality and Social Psychology*, 61, pp. 776-788.

Sears, D.O. (1983), 'The person-positivity bias', *Journal of Personality and Social Psychology*, 44, pp. 233-250.

Slovic, P., Fischhoff, B. and Lichtenstein, S. (1978), 'Accident probabilities and seat belt usage: a psychological perspective', *Accident Analysis and Prevention*, 10, pp. 281-285.

Svenson, O. (1981), 'Are we all less risky and more skillful than our fellow drivers?', *Acta Psychologica*, 47, pp. 143-148.

Svenson, O., Fischhoff, B. and MacGregor, D. (1985), 'Perceived driving safety and seatbelt usage', *Accident Analysis and Prevention*, 17, pp. 119-133.

Taylor, S.E. and Brown, J.D. (1988), 'Illusion and well-being: a social psychological perspective on mental health', *Psychological Bulletin*, 103, pp. 193-210.

Tyler, T.R. and Cook, F.L. (1994), 'The mass media and judgments of risk: distinguishing impact on personal and societal level judgments', *Journal of Personality and Social Psychology*, 47, pp. 693-708.

Van der Pligt, J. (1991), 'Risicoperceptie, onrealistisch optimisme en AIDS-preventief gedrag', *Nederlands Tijdschrift voor de Psychologie*, 46, pp. 228-237.

Van der Velde, F.W., Hooijkaas, C. and Van der Pligt, J (1991), 'Risk perception and behavior: pessimism, realism, and optimism about AIDS-related health behavior', *Psychology and Health*, 6, pp. 23-38.

Weinstein, N.D. (1980), 'Unrealistic optimism about future life events', *Journal of Personality and Social Psychology*, 39, pp. 806-820.

Weinstein, N.D. (1982), 'Unrealistic optimism about susceptibility to health problems', *Journal of Behavioral Medicine*, 5, pp. 441-460.

Weinstein, N.D. (1983), 'Reducing unrealistic optimism about illness susceptibility', *Health Psychology*, 2, pp. 11-20.

Weinstein, N.D. (1984), 'Why it won't happen to me: perceptions of risk factors and susceptibility', *Health Psychology*, 3, pp. 431-437.

Weinstein, N.D. (1987), 'Unrealistic optimism about susceptibility to health problems: conclusions from a community-wide sample', *Journal of Behavioral Medicine*, 10, pp. 481-500.
Weinstein, N.D. (1988), 'The precaution adoption process', *Health Psychology*, 7, pp. 355-386.
Weinstein, N.D. (1989), 'Optimistic biases about personal risks', *Science*, 246, pp. 1232-1233.
Weinstein, N.D., Grubb, P.D. and Vautier, J. (1986), 'Increasing automobile seatbelt use: an intervention emphasizing risk susceptibility', *Journal of Applied Psychology*, 71, pp. 285-290.
Weinstein, N.D., Klotz, M.L. and Sandman, P.M. (1988), 'Optimistic biases in public perceptions of the risk from radon', *American Journal of Public Health*, 178, pp. 796-800.
Weinstein, N.D. and Lachendro, E. (1982), 'Egocentrism as a source of unrealistic optimism', *Personality and Social Psychology Bulletin*, 8, pp. 195-200.
Weinstein, N.D., Sandman, P.M. and Roberts, N.E. (1990), 'Determinants of self-protective behavior: home radon testing', *Journal of Applied Social Psychology*, 20, pp. 783-801.
Wood, J.V. (1989), 'Theory and research concerning social comparisons of personal attributes', *Psychological Bulletin*, 106, pp. 231-248.
Zakay, D. (1983), 'The relationship between the probability assessor and the outcomes of an event as a determiner of subjective probability', *Acta Psychologica*, 53, pp. 271-280.
Zakay, D. (1984), 'The influence of a perceived event's controllability on its subjective occurrence probability', *Psychological Record*, 34, pp. 233-240.

9 The development of AIDS education for Dutch secondary schools: A systematic approach based on theory, research and cooperation

H.P. Schaalma, G. Kok, J. Poelman and J. Reinders

When developing health education one is confronted with a variety of decisions regarding the content of the educational message, the target groups, the media, and so on. Unfortunately, these decisions cannot be made on the basis of some cookery book for health education: they have to be based on previous theoretical or empirical work. The only 'rule' is that the effectiveness of the education is dependent on the quality of the planning process (Mullen, Green and Persinger, 1985; Green and Kreuter, 1991). Health education should be based on a diagnosis of the behaviour in question, of the psychosocial behavioural determinants, and of the options for an intervention. Furthermore, interventions should be systematically evaluated.

Perhaps one of the most difficult steps is the translation of knowledge about behavioural determinants into feasible interventions using current fundamental insights from the behavioural sciences, especially social psychology, sociology and communication sciences. The present chapter addresses this issue, describing the systematic development of AIDS education for Dutch secondary schools. Special attention will be paid to a spiral approach to data gathering in which qualitative and quantitative methods are combined (De Vries et al., 1992), and to the need for cooperation between researchers, practical workers, teachers and students (Kok and Green, 1991).

Determinants of safe sex

Before 1990 there were very few studies of the determinants of safe sex behaviours among Dutch youth (Schaalma et al., 1991). We therefore devised and set up a programme of research, to be based on a version of the Theory of Planned Behaviour (Ajzen, 1991). Three determinants of behaviour were distinguished (Figure 9.1): attitudes towards the behaviour, and beliefs concerning the consequences of the behaviour (Fishbein and Ajzen, 1975); beliefs about social norms (Fishbein and Ajzen, 1975), the behaviour of others (Bandura, 1986), or social expectations and social pressure (Suls and Wills, 1991); and beliefs about control (Ajzen, 1991), self-efficacy (Bandura, 1986), or success expectancy (Weiner, 1986). The determinants may be seen as both behavioural antecedents and behavioural consequences (Zimbardo and Leippe, 1991).

First, a survey of the literature about young people's contraception and AIDS prevention and about theoretical and empirical work on smoking behaviour was conducted — to provide initial ideas about the determinants of safe(r) sex. To highlight and broaden those ideas, the second step in our research made use of group interviews with students guided by a professional youth worker, and other interviews with youth workers, local health educators, and teachers. Finally, a questionnaire was developed concerning the determinants of two safe sex behaviours: condom use and sex without intercourse. The questionnaire also addressed AIDS knowledge and risk perception.

The questionnaire was pretested by means of group interviews with students to assess comprehensibility, length, and language, and by means of a survey of a further 207 students (mean age 15.8 years). Besides several practical issues, the survey revealed that attitudes, perceived social norms, and self-efficacy expectations concerning condom use were more positive than attitudes, norms, and self-efficacy expectations concerning sex without intercourse. Consequently, the students' intention to use condoms was significantly higher than their intention to have sex without intercourse.

The results of the interviews and survey suggest that AIDS education should principally advocate condom use. Advocating sex without intercourse does not seem to be a realistic option for AIDS education because of the high discrepancy between the message and students' current attitudes (McGuire, 1985). Besides, students may not receive social support for practising sex without intercourse (Brownell et al., 1986), and education should not advocate behaviour of which students have low self-efficacy expectations (Locke and Latham, 1991). Of course, differences between groups of students are important for deciding the message to be advocated by AIDS education — for example, differences between boys and girls (Richard and Van der Pligt, 1991; Schaalma, Kok and Peters, 1993a), or between ethnic groups (Vogels and Van der Vliet, 1990) — for groups may differ in their knowledge, values, attitudes, skills, and social contexts (Flora and Thoresen, 1988). Intervention programmes should take such differences into consideration, and should be tailored to specific groups, or made suitable for use with heterogeneous groups.

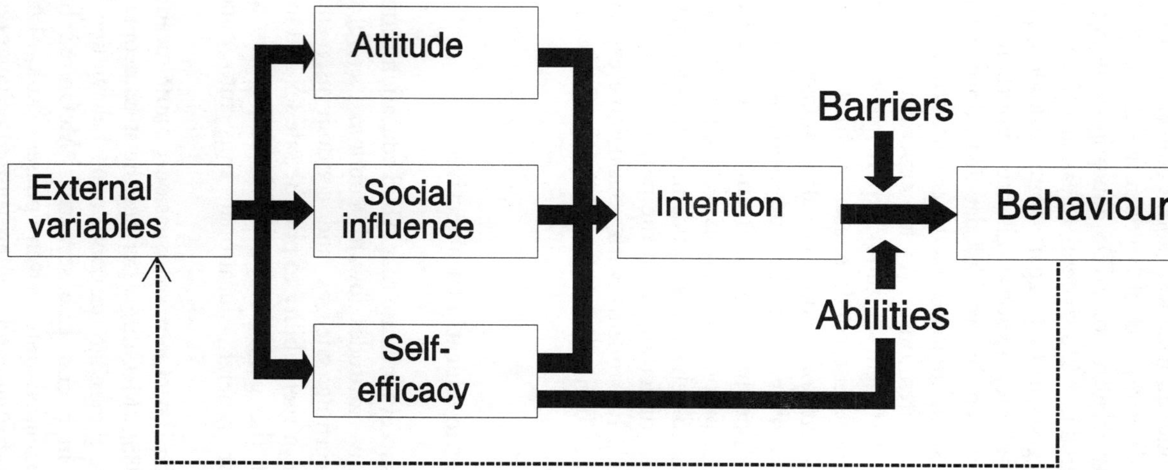

Figure 9.1 Model of determinants of behaviour

A second study addressed the impact of behavioural experience on the determinants of consistent condom use (see also Schaalma et al., 1993a). Experience of intercourse may affect beliefs about condom use, about social pressures (Fishbein and Ajzen, 1975), and about self-efficacy (Bandura, 1990), but information about the impact of behavioural experience on the determinants of condom use is sparse, even though it may be particularly relevant for AIDS education. A questionnaire was therefore administered to 1,018 students (mean age 15.1 years). The results confirmed the suggestion that, apart from attitudes, perceived social influences and self-efficacy expectations are important determinants of intended condom use, and it provided detailed information about beliefs and expectations that differentiated students with positive intentions from those with negative intentions. As for experience of intercourse, the results indicated that students without experience generally had positive attitudes towards consistent condom use, but that there was a marked decline in the popularity of condom use after students had begun having sexual intercourse. Furthermore, the study showed that students did not perceive consistent condom use as the norm among themselves and their peers, and that a large proportion were expecting problems with consistent condom use and related behaviours. Students without experience were the most likely to expect difficulties with the purchase of condoms and with carrying them regularly; students with considerable experience were the most likely to expect difficulties in maintaining consistent use within a steady relationship.

From determinants to educational objectives

The results of the surveys indicate that AIDS education should (a) enhance and reinforce positive attitudes towards condom use; (b) create positive social norms concerning safe sex and condom use; and (c) enhance students' self-belief in their ability to practise safe sex and to use condoms. The next step in the programme's development was a theory-based translation of our general educational aims into concrete, specific objectives.

As a theoretical basis McGuire's Persuasion-Communication Matrix was used (McGuire, 1985). McGuire describes the steps people take from the initial response, to a message, to continuous behavioural change in the desired direction, in a best case scenario. McGuire's framework was simplified and extended into seven phases (Kok, 1991): successful communication (*attention* and *comprehension*); changes in behavioural determinants (*attitude*, *social influence*, *self-efficacy*) and *behaviour*; and *maintenance* of behaviour change. Interventions may be different for each step, and the decisions that have to be made about the message, the channel, the source, and the target group may be different too and may even conflict. Within the framework a variety of theories can be applied — theories that may cover only (parts of) specific steps in the process of behaviour change, but that can be helpful when developing interventions.

Successful communication

School based AIDS education may reduce the problems of selective exposure and selective attention (McGuire, 1985). However, most students seem to regard themselves as personally invulnerable (Abrams et al., 1990), and not all of them will be interested in AIDS education — perhaps because of unrealistic optimism (Weinstein, 1989, and Hoorens in this volume). The probable reasons are an underestimation of what others do to protect themselves, and a stereotypical image of high risk groups. Risk information may be personalized by providing information about the protective behaviour of similar others, by emphasizing risky behaviour instead of risk groups, and by providing scenario-based risk information (Hendrickx, 1991).

Students' attention may further be enhanced by a positive, personalized message, and by attractive and appealing methods and materials. The message should be geared to their level of sexual development: AIDS education for lower grade students should be organized around starting sexual relationships, while in the higher grades it should address AIDS prevention in the context of 'steady' relationships. The programme should use appealing media methods, such as videos and popular TV programmes, teen magazines, and active participation. It should use attractive sources, such as peers and popular referents. To enhance attraction and comprehension, the programme should be tailored to students' language and to their priorities and values, taking into account differences between gender groups, ethnic groups, educational level, and so on (Bunton, Murphy and Bennett, 1991). The message should be easy to understand and well organized, and repetition and explicit conclusions may be useful (Burgoon, 1989). Written materials added to video and class activities may also enhance comprehension, and it should be remembered that peers are important sources for translating expert knowledge into comprehensive information. Furthermore, teaching methods based on active learning and active participation will enhance elaboration of the message, and consequently comprehension (Petty and Cacioppo, 1986).

Attitude change

In order to enhance or reinforce positive attitudes towards condom use, education should first of all increase and reinforce students' knowledge about AIDS. From the perspective of preventing discrimination against AIDS patients, misconceptions about the possibility of contracting AIDS by daily interactions (e.g. sharing bathrooms) deserve special attention (Schaalma, Peters and Kok, 1993b). Attitudes can be changed by presenting new information, and by enhancing the salience of information already possessed (McGuire, 1985). The 'Socratic Method' of teaching, a method in which questioning is used to elicit information, is preferable to the didactic approach because it reduces resistance to the message and encourages discussion and consensus among group members (see for example Flay et al., 1988). To enhance the persuasiveness of the message, sources have to be attractive, competent and reliable (McGuire, 1985). A combination of experts, teachers and peers may be most effective. Communication theory does not provide clear suggestions for other factors that may affect the persuasiveness of a message, such as organizational structure, ordering of arguments, logic, number of arguments, explicitness of conclusions, and repetition of message components (Burgoon, 1989).

Education should increase the salience of the personal advantages of condom use and the personal disadvantages of unprotected intercourse. Short term advantages and disadvantages are preferable because they are most salient (McGuire, 1985). Because most students accept the preventive advantages of using condoms (Schaalma et al., 1993a), it seems worth trying to emphasize additional short term advantages, such as the lower chance of early ejaculation, the avoidance of messy postcoital discharge of semen from the vagina (Hatcher and Sammons Hughes, 1988), and the prevention of feelings of regret (Richard and Van der Pligt, 1991). A two sided message acknowledging the advantages and disadvantages of condom use may be preferable because most students will have been, or soon will be, exposed to arguments opposing safe sex (Burgoon, 1989). Theories about risk perception (e.g. Kahneman, Slovic and Tversky, 1986) and fear-arousing communications (R.W. Rogers, 1983; Leventhal, 1984; Janz and Becker, 1984) suggest that increasing fear by emphasizing the 'losses' of unsafe sex may also be a motivator for practising safe(r) sex, on condition that it is accompanied by adequate suggestions for coping with the fear. It may also be possible to stimulate positive reactions to condoms by repeated exposure, by associating condom use with other positive stimuli (Zimbardo and Leippe, 1991), and by means of erotic instructions (Tanner and Pollack, 1988). The programme should not give the impression that practising safe sex is something unpleasant. The discrepancy between students' current attitudes and behaviour and the advocated behaviour should not be too large (McGuire, 1985). AIDS education should therefore start before students have begun to have sexual intercourse. Because the current attitudes towards condom use among students without experience are relatively positive, naive students may be the most receptive.

Social support

Social Comparison Theory assumes that people tend to conform to the attitudes and behaviour of similar others, partly because those others provide information about social reality, and partly because conformity may be socially rewarding (Suls and Wills, 1991). Young people, however, communicate very little about sexuality and AIDS prevention, and most of them have only vague ideas about what their peers think and do. AIDS education should clarify perceptions of group norms about safe sex by providing information about the way peers respond to questions about sexuality and AIDS prevention, and by enhancing communication. The possible role for parents in AIDS education is unclear. It may be worthwhile to include parents in a prevention programme (Schaalma et al., 1993a), but involving parents and increasing parent-child communication about sexual topics may be very difficult (Kirby et al., 1991).

Research on group polarization has shown that group discussion may strengthen the initial position of the group members (Isenberg, 1986). If the average pre-discussion position of the group favours unsafe sex, group discussion may lead to a 'risky shift' — because of the exchange of arguments favouring the pre-discussion position, and because of social comparison of views. Teachers should be alert to the possibility of shifts in favour of unsafe sex, and may have to stop group discussions when the majority of students strongly favour it. Teachers may also help to prevent undesired shifts by supporting arguments and views that favour safe sex, and by presenting support from other reference groups.

A useful strategy for dealing with social pressure to practise unsafe sex is to enhance students' refusal skills. Skills training based on psychological inoculation (McGuire, 1964), social inoculation (Evans, Getz and Raines, 1991), vicarious learning, and modelling (Bandura, 1986) may improve students' abilities to cope with sexuality and AIDS prevention. Training should (a) provide students with counterarguments; (b) show models resisting social pressures, preferably peers (e.g. Clarke et al., 1986); (c) anchor beliefs in favour of safe sex to important values (e.g. life goals), other beliefs (e.g. being responsible), or admired others; (d) enhance students' assertiveness (cf. De Vries and Kok, 1986), and (e) give practice in applying information and skills in troublesome situations (Gilchrist and Schinke, 1983).

Self-efficacy improvement

Social Learning Theory (Bandura, 1986) suggests that people learn new behaviour by observing other people, and by observing the consequences of their own behaviour. Students' self-belief in their ability to practise safe(r) sex may thus be enhanced by mastery experience, vicarious learning, and/or social persuasion (Bandura, 1990). To increase their self-belief about condom use and related skills, students need encouragement and successful experiences with the purchase of condoms, carrying them on dates, negotiating their use, and using them adequately (Basen-Engquist and Parcel, 1992; Schaalma et al., 1993a). Bandura (1986) suggests a learning process in which four phases can be distinguished: breaking up complex behaviour into subskills that are easier to handle; modelling to facilitate comprehension of the behaviour; guided enactment of the behaviour in easy situations, followed by feedback; and guided enactment of the behaviour in more difficult situations, followed by feedback. A combination of modelling and role playing seems to be an effective strategy to enhance skills (Gilchrist and Schinke, 1983), and adequate feedback and reinforcement provided by teachers may be essential elements in the acquisition of skills. In the classroom, skills training about safe sex is limited to behaviours that are related to the actual sexual behaviour, such as decision making, communication, and resisting social pressures. To compensate, the programme should include materials that explicitly demonstrate how to use condoms and how to handle real life troublesome situations — by means of cartoons, computer animations, or video, for example.

Behaviour change and maintenance

Because a school based programme for AIDS prevention cannot provide feedback on actual sexual behaviour, it should stimulate students to communicate about sexual matters and AIDS prevention with people who might provide feedback, such as school counsellors, experts at STD clinics, AIDS hotlines, etc. Some behaviours related to AIDS prevention, however, can be practised within the context of a school curriculum, for example purchasing condoms, carrying them regularly, and negotiating their use. Practising safe(r) sex may also be stimulated by 'prompts' that remind students of their intentions (Zimbardo and Leippe, 1991), and by repeated expressions of positive attitudes (Fazio, 1986), for example by means of posters and stickers. To enhance behaviour maintenance, the programme should also include 'booster' sessions (Flay, 1985), if possible continuing throughout the student's school career.

Situations that interfere with intentions to practise safe sex, and negative experiences of practising it, may produce lapses into unsafe sex. Current health education emphasizes the enhancement of self-efficacy to prevent and overcome possible lapses (Den Boer et al., 1991), using Attribution Theory (Weiner, 1986) and Relapse-Prevention Theory (Marlatt and Gordon, 1985). Students who attribute lapsing to external and uncontrollable causes will need to be convinced that they have control over practising safe sex, and that they need to improve their skills or to try harder. According to relapse prevention theory, students should be taught how to cope with interfering situations and experiences, for example by means of forewarning and pre-exposure. Theories about economic decision making suggest that anticipated regret of specific behavioural alternatives determines behavioural choice (e.g. Loomes and Sugden, 1982). Anticipating negative affective reactions may help students to prevent lapses (Richard and Van der Pligt, 1991).

According to Goal Setting Theory (Locke and Latham, 1991), setting a challenging goal may result in a better performance than setting an easy goal or no goal at all, provided that the relevant abilities and self-efficacy, goal commitment, goal acceptance, and feedback, are present. Setting goals in life may enhance students' motivation to avoid unsafe sex and to overcome relapse, as long as they recognize the correspondence between their present behaviour and their goals.

From educational objectives to a curriculum

The next step in the developing process consists of the translation of theoretical ideas into practical teaching methods and materials. Although there is extensive knowledge of teaching methods and activities that are frequently used in school based primary prevention projects (Sussman, 1991), little is known about the effectiveness and practicability of specific teaching methods. Curriculum developers can overcome the knowledge gap (a) by developing their programmes in collaboration with teachers, educational experts, and students; (b) by carefully pretesting methods and materials (Kok and Green, 1990); and (c) by diagnosing teachers' wishes, needs and abilities.

When developing AIDS education programmes one should also take into account political and religious barriers to smooth diffusion. The school system that is expected to adopt and implement the curriculum should be invited and encouraged to participate from an early stage (Kok and Green, 1990). One approach is to include representatives of both the developers and the school system, together with change agents who facilitate collaboration, in an attempt to bridge the gap that often remains when innovation-development barriers and diffusion barriers are considered separately (Orlandi et al., 1990).

Diagnosis of the school system

Dutch secondary schools can be categorized by religious affiliation and by educational level. Although most of the AIDS education programmes that have been developed for different school types are similar with respect to goals and methods, one should take into account possible differences in norms and values when developing new programmes. As an illustration, one organization of religious schools refused to distribute an AIDS curriculum because of what it saw as a one sided emphasis on condom use. It was therefore decided (a) to embed AIDS prevention in the broader context of relationship formation, and (b) to pay attention to the prevailing norms and values regarding sexuality and related matters.

It was also decided to tailor the new curriculum to students of vocational schools and schools for lower general secondary education. Students in these schools have relatively little knowledge about AIDS, and on average they start having (unsafe) sex at an early age (Vogels and Van der Vliet, 1990). Moreover, the proportion of such schools that provide AIDS education is low when compared to other schools (Paulussen and Bartels, 1992). Although about 85 per cent of Dutch secondary schools provide some AIDS education, most of the teachers have low self-efficacy expectations regarding skill oriented teaching methods, and few of them use methods such as role playing (Paulussen and Bartels, 1992). A needs assessment among teachers about a smoking prevention programme revealed that new curricula need not require special time consuming training (De Vries et al., 1992).

Programme development

In order to introduce some kind of skills training for AIDS prevention in the Dutch school system, it was decided to develop a curriculum in which the skills part of the programme was structured by video. Interactive video is well suited to social modelling, and is an effective means of increasing students' knowledge and skills. Video provides opportunities (a) to show the process of social influence and conformity, (b) to introduce positive role models into the classroom, and (c) to demonstrate dialogues about safe sex in lifelike high risk situations. Furthermore, video may facilitate the introduction of skills training by means of role playing techniques without the need for time consuming teacher training sessions: role playing can be structured, exercises can be introduced, and feedback can be provided.

The video we have developed deals with young people's beliefs and values concerning safe sex, reasons for having unsafe sex, perceived barriers to practising it, communication about it, and standing up to pressures against practising it. The first part presents a group of young people making a television programme for a local broadcasting company. They are shown interviewing peers about safe sex, and discussing the interviews during the production sessions. The video also presents a girl demonstrating condom use on her boyfriend's fingers, as well as a computer animation. Figure 9.2 presents a further excerpt — an interview scene in which a girl talks about unsafe sex on holiday. The second part of the video presents four scenes, all concerned with standing up to social pressures. First, a lifelike situation is introduced, for example one in which a boy is pressing his girlfriend to have intercourse. Halfway through the dialogue, the teacher stops the video tape, and students are asked to finish the dialogue in subgroups, discussing specific questions — after which the video finishes with a happy ending. The dialogues, the viewing exercise, and the teacher's instructions for the discussions are all based on social inoculation (e.g. Evans et al., 1991) and are intended to help students build their resistance to social pressure against safe sex: (1) say what you want, (2) think about the arguments, (3) stick to your opinion, (4) present alternatives, (5) give counter pressure, and, if that does not work, (6) walk away (avoidance). Figure 9.3 presents an outline of one of the scenes.

Apart from the video, the curriculum includes three further sets of material: a teacher manual which discusses teaching objectives, materials, methods and operations, and provides background information; a teen magazine which presents information about AIDS and other STDs and how to prevent them, and discusses attitudes and values about sexual matters; and recall material linking up with the national campaign 'Safe sex on holiday'. A variety of exercises are also provided, to enhance the flexibility of the programme. Throughout, the central teaching principles are active participation and social modelling. Apart from 'Socratic teaching', the curriculum includes a variety of writing exercises, homework assignments, small group activities and discussions, and viewing exercises. For example, students are asked to monitor and assess the opinions of others about safe sex, by watching the video and completing a checklist. As well as facts about AIDS and other STDs, the student magazine

A Holiday Affair

The video shows a boy and girl, both about 15 years old, being interviewed about safe sex. The girl talks about her last holiday. Despite good intentions she had given in to a holiday lover pressing her to have intercourse without a condom.

'Last year I had a holiday affair. Of course, we ended up in bed. I wanted to practise safe sex, and brought condoms along, but he didn't want to use one. And he kept on pushing ... Stupid. But he was such a gorgeous piece, I couldn't let him go. Besides, he looked very neat. I was stupid, and we had sex without a condom. I use the pill, you know ... During the next few days I was in a terrible panic. And of course, I had discharge ... an STD. Chlamydia. It scared the hell out of me. It can make you infertile.'

With her current boyfriend she had made a deal about having safe sex: she takes care of the pill, he takes care of condoms.

Figure 9.2

Rene and Irene

The situation:
Rene and Irene, both about 15 years old, are watching television at Rene's place. Rene's parents are out for the evening. They hesitantly make advances to each other, and start to fondle and kiss. Rene wants to have intercourse (with a condom). Irene, however, does not want to go that far.

The viewing exercise:
Irene likes Rene a lot, and does not want to lose him.
How can she explain to Rene that she likes him a lot, but that she does not want to have sexual intercourse yet?
How would Rene react?
And how will it end?

The happy ending:
Although Rene persists, Irene manages to cope with the situation by backing up her opinion with arguments, by presenting alternatives (fondling, kissing), by providing counter-pressure, and by rewarding Rene ('I like your kisses.')

Figure 9.3

Condom use

Condom use? Are there any disadvantages? When you ask young people this question, they are quick with their opinions. Jeroen, for example, says: 'With a rubber you don't feel anything'. According to Tarik, that's way over the top: 'Bullshit, a rubber is so thin that you'll hardly notice it. Jeroen has probably never even tried it!'. According to Ewout, however, Jeroen is partly right. With a rubber you may feel less, but that's rather an advantage. 'You won't come so fast; making love will last longer!'.

Figure 9.4

Source: Dutch STD Foundation (1992), *Long Live Love: What You Need to Know about Aids and Other STDs*

provides information about attitudes and values regarding sexual matters and AIDS prevention, through short statements and vignettes that present peer models talking about their values, attitudes, expectations, problems, and experiences. Figure 9.4 presents an example, and Figure 9.5 provides an overview of the whole curriculum.

Pretest and participation

An essential element in curriculum development is pretesting, for it allows the reactions of experts and members of the target population to be gauged at an early stage in a programme's life. A pretest is generally valuable to test an intervention's attractiveness, comprehensibility, relevance, credibility, acceptability, undesired side effects, and workability. The need for pretesting is strongest when (a) little is known about the target population, (b) the content of the programme is controversial, and (c) money is at stake (Damoiseaux, 1991).

Our own curriculum was pretested by means of interviews with teachers and educational experts. The interviews addressed the suitability and feasibility of the teaching methods, and examined expectations about how long preparation and instruction would take. Our original attempt was shown to be too radical, and the discrepancy between proposed teaching methods and usual methods was shown to be too large. Consequently, the curriculum was revised and a variety of methods currently in use were included in the final version.

The student magazine was first pretested on 147 students, who completed a questionnaire that addressed the layout of the pages and the attractiveness of the illustrations. Generally, the magazine was evaluated positively: 79 per cent of the students liked it; 54 per cent liked the illustrations; 69 per cent found it well organized; and 88 per cent liked the balance between text and illustrations. In a second pretest, the comprehensibility and persuasiveness of the magazine were tested on 119 students, using a pre-test post-test control group design. Respondents completed a knowledge questionnaire, and were asked to evaluate the magazine's quality, clarity, usefulness, newsworthiness, and closeness to real life. Both pretests led us to make changes to the magazine, in content and style.

A synopsis of the video was pretested by means of two group interviews with students. Respondents evaluated the ideas the video contained and provided suggestions for translating the synopsis into a scenario. A model scenario was pretested among 44 students, using content response coding (US DHHS, 1984), and the off-line montage was previewed by 83 students who assessed it for attractiveness, credibility, and closeness to real life.

Objectives	Theoretical underpinnings	Methods/materials
■ Enhancement of knowledge and risk perception ■ Attitude change/ reinforcement	(Social) learning theory; communication theory (attention, comprehension, discrepancy, repetition, time gap, clear conclusions); elaboration likelihood; risk perception (fear arousal; unrealistic optimism; scenario-based information); outcome expectancies; discrepancy; affective response; social comparison (group polarization); psychological inoculation	Classes: 'Socratic' teaching, reading exercises, group discussions, small group assignments, homework, quiz, test Magazine: attractive design (colours, illustrations); information (facts, values, attitudes) provided by peer models (vignettes); assignments and exercises (writing, interviews) Video: appealing production and design (music, graphics); information provided by peer models
■ Clarifying/ enhancing norms ■ Improving refusal skills	Social learning theory (modelling, enactive learning, feedback) Social comparison, conformity Social inoculation	Classes: 'Socratic' teaching, group discussion, homework assignments (writing exercises, interviews), and viewing exercise Magazine: peer models regarding resisting social pressure Video: peer models (positive attitudes, resisting social pressure, practising safe sex; solving problems)
■ Enhancement of self-efficacy	Social learning theory (modelling, enactive learning, feedback)	Classes: group discussions, viewing exercise regarding solving troublesome situations, homework assignment (purchase of condoms; use), demonstration of condom use Magazine: peer models (vignettes) regarding solving problems with putting condom use into practice (buying, taking along, talking about) Video: computer animation of condom use; presentation of troublesome situations, feedback
■ Maintenance	Relapse prevention (forewarning, pre-exposure); anticipated affect; goal setting; commitment; learning theory (prompts; repeated exposure)	Classes: short rehearsal at the end of the school year, reinforcement of good intentions, attractive brochure 'Safe sex on holiday', posters, sticker

Figure 9.5 AIDS education for secondary schools: objectives, theoretical underpinnings, methods, and materials

Again pretesting led to changes. A student panel was also frequently consulted during the later development of the programme.

Linkage

To bridge the gap between research and development on the one hand and the school system on the other, a linkage board was set up. The board was made up of representatives from the research and development group, the school advisory services, and the organizations that provide sex and AIDS education to secondary schools. A member of the development team acted as change agent. The role of the board was to provide feedback about the main principles underlying the curriculum, and to give advice on implementation and diffusion.

Conclusions

Although it is too early to tell whether the programme we have outlined will affect students' sexual behaviour, the systematic approach to curriculum development appears to be sound. The combination of literature survey, interviews and a carefully pretested questionnaire proved to be a useful approach for gathering data. The literature searches and interviews provided information about students' most salient beliefs about AIDS prevention and condom use, which was then used for constructing the questionnaire. The questionnaire was pretested by means of interviews and a small survey, and provided comprehensive data about the determinants of condom use and related behaviours. It also gave us detailed information about the gaps in students' knowledge, and about the psychosocial determinants of condom use as a means of preventing AIDS.

The systematic application of theory, using a framework of persuasion, proved to be useful as well. McGuire's Persuasion-Communication Matrix (1985) was helpful for the translation of theory into practice, and a variety of theories provided guiding ideas for the curriculum and its components. The matrix helped us not only to choose the message, the target group, the channels and the sources, but also to apply the theories.

The participation of teachers, curriculum specialists and students was a further important part of the design process, for the various pretests and advisory panels produced valuable feedback. Moreover, the combination of quantitative and qualitative methods proved to be especially useful: quantitative research provided detailed information about teachers' specific needs and wishes, and about the persuasive impact of the student magazine; qualitative research provided feedback about the workability of the curriculum, the possible barriers to its implementation, and the attractiveness and validity of the materials. A full scale evaluation of the curriculum should provide further information: quantitative methods should be used for assessing the effectiveness and fidelity of the programme, while qualitative methods should be able to provide further information about its workability.

The formation of a linkage board for helping innovation, development, and diffusion seems to be a useful step for bridging the gap between research, development and the school system. However, a linkage board is no guarantee of smooth diffusion, and a variety of additional steps will need to be taken. In particular, future research will have to examine what helps and what hinders the dissemination of health education curricula. Diffusion theory (E.M. Rogers, 1983), social learning theory (Bandura, 1986), and theories about organizational change (Goodman and Steckler, 1990) should all provide useful leads.

Acknowledgements

Our research is supported by funds from the Dutch Ministry of Welfare, Health and Cultural Affairs (grant no. 90020). The authors wish to thank Ruud Coolen and Louk Peters for their contribution to the development of the curriculum, and Henk Aarts and Monique Mensen for their contribution to the research.

References

Abrams, D., Abraham, C., Spears, R. and Marks, D. (1990), 'AIDS invulnerability: relationships, sexual behaviour and attitudes among 16-19-year-olds', in Aggleton, P., Davies, P. and Hart, G. (eds), *AIDS. Individual, Cultural and Policy Dimensions*, The Falmer Press, London, pp. 35-52.

Ajzen, I. (1991), 'The Theory of Planned Behavior', *Organizational Behavior and Human Decision Processes*, 50, pp. 179-211.

Bandura, A. (1986), *Social Foundations of Thought and Action: A Social Cognitive Theory*, Prentice Hall, Englewood Cliffs, NJ.

Bandura, A. (1990), Perceived self-efficacy in the exercise of control over AIDS-infection, *Evaluation and Programme Planning*, 13, pp. 9-17.

Basen-Engquist, K. and Parcel, G.S. (1992), 'Attitudes, norms and self-efficacy: a model of adolescents' HIV-related sexual risk behavior', *Health Education Quarterly*, 19, pp. 263-277.

Brownell, K.D., Marlatt, G.A., Lichtenstein, E. and Wilson, G.T. (1986), 'Understanding and preventing relapse', *American Psychologist*, 41, pp. 756-782.

Bunton, R., Murphy, S., Bennett, P. (1991), 'Theories of behavioural change and their use in health promotion: some neglected areas', *Health Education Research*, 6, pp. 153-162.

Burgoon, M. (1989), 'Messages and persuasive effects: review of issues in message-effects research in the social influence literature', in Bradac, J.J. (ed.), *Message Effects in Communication Science*, Sage Publications, Newbury Park, pp. 129-164.

Clarke, J.H., MacPherson, B., Holmes, D.R. and Jones, R. (1986), 'Reducing adolescent smoking: a comparison of peer-led, teacher-led, and expert intervention', *Journal of Consulting and Clinical Psychology*, 53, pp. 102-106.

Damoiseaux, V. (1991), *Advantages and Disadvantages of Mass Communication* (in Dutch), Van Gorcum, Assen/Maastricht.

Den Boer, D-J., Kok, G., Hospers, H.J., Gerards, F.M., Strecher, V.J. (1991), 'Health education strategies for attributional retraining and self-efficacy improvement', *Health Education Research*, 6, pp. 239-248.

De Vries, H. and Kok, G. (1986), 'From determinants of smoking behaviour to the implications for a smoking prevention programme', *Health Education Research*, 1 (2), pp. 85-94.

De Vries, H., Weijts, W., Dijkstra, M. and Kok, G. (1992), 'The utilization of qualitative and quantitative data for health education planning, implementation and evaluation: a spiral approach', *Health Education Quarterly*, 19 (1), pp. 101-115.

Evans, R.I., Getz, J.G. and Raines, B.E. (1991), 'Theory guided models on prevention of AIDS in adolescents', paper presented at the Science Weekend at the American Psychological Association Meeting, 16-20 August 1991, San Francisco, California.

Fazio, R.H. (1986), 'How do attitudes guide behavior?', in Sorentino, R.M. and Higgins, E.T. (eds), *The Handbook of Motivation and Cognition*, New York, Guilford.

Fishbein, M. and Ajzen, I. (1975), *Belief, Attitude, Intention and Behavior: An Introduction to Theory and Research*, Addison Wesley, Reading, Mass.

Flay, B.R. (1985), 'Psychosocial approaches to smoking prevention: a review of findings', *Health Psychology*, 4 (5), pp. 449-488.

Flay, B.R., Brannon, B.R., Johnson, C.A., Hansen, W.B., Ulene, A.L., Whitney-Saltiel, D.A., Gleason, L.R., Sussman, S., Gavin, M., Glowacz, K.M., Sobol, D.F. and Spiegel, D.C. (1988), 'The television, school, and family smoking prevention/cessation project: I. Theoretical basis and program development', *Preventive Medicine*, 17, pp. 585-607.

Flora, J.A. and Thoresen, C.E. (1988), 'Reducing the risk of AIDS in adolescents', *American Psychologist*, 43 (11), pp. 965-970.
Gilchrist, L.D., and Schinke, S.P. (1983), 'Coping with contraception: cognitive and behavioral methods with adolescents', *Cognitive Therapy and Research*, 7, pp. 379-388.
Goodman, R.M. and Steckler, A.B. (1990), 'Mobilizing organizations for health enhancement: theories of organizational change', in Glanz, K, Lewis, F.M. and Rimer, B. (eds), *Health Behavior and Health Education: Theory, Research and Practice*, Jossey-Bass, San Francisco, CA.
Green, L.W and Kreuter, M.W. (1991), *Health Promotion Planning: An Educational and Environmental Approach*, Second Edition, Mayfield Publishing Company, Mountain View.
Hatcher, R.A. and Sammons Hughes, M. (1988), 'The truth about condoms', *Siecus Report*, 17, (2), pp. 88-95.
Hendrickx, L. (1991), *How Versus How Often*, Van Denderen, Groningen.
Howard, M. and McCabe, J.B. (1990), 'Helping teenagers postpone sexual involvement', *Family Planning Perspectives*, 22, pp. 21-26.
Isenberg, D.J. (1986), 'Group polarization: a critical review and meta analysis', *Journal of Personality and Social Psychology*, 50, pp. 1141-1151.
Janz, N.K. and Becker, M.H. (1989), 'The Health Belief Model: a decade later', *Health Education Quarterly*, 11, pp. 1-47.
Kahneman, D., Slovic, P. and Tversky, A. (1986), *Judgement Under Uncertainty: Heuristics and Biases*, Cambridge University Press, Cambridge.
Kirby, D., Barth, R.P., Leland, N. and Fetro, J.V. (1991), 'Reducing the Risk: impact of a new curriculum on sexual risk-taking', *Family Planning Perspectives*, 23 (6), pp. 253-263.
Kirby, D., Waszak, C. and Ziegler, J. (1991), 'Six school-based clinics: their reproductive health services and impact on sexual behavior', *Family Planning Perspectives*, 23 (1), pp. 6-16.
Kok, G.J. (1991), 'Health education theories and research for AIDS prevention', *Hygie*, 10, pp. 32-39.
Kok, G. and Green, L.W. (1990), 'Research to support health promotion in practice: a plea for increased co-operation', *Health Promotion International*, 5 (4), pp. 303-308.
Leventhal, H. (1984), 'A perceptual-motor theory of emotion', in Berkowitz, L. (ed.), *Advances in Experimental Social Psychology*, Vol. 17, Academic Press, New York.
Locke, E.A. and Latham, G.P. (1991), *A Theory of Goal Setting and Task Performance*, Prentice Hall, Englewood Cliffs, NJ.
Loomes, G. and Sugden, R. (1982), 'Regret Theory: an alternative theory of rational choice under uncertainty', *Economic Journal*, 92, pp. 805-825.

Marlatt, G.A. and Gordon, J.R. (1985), *Relapse Prevention: Maintenance Strategies in the Treatment of Addictive Behaviors*, Guilford, New York.
McGuire, L.W. (1964), 'Inducing resistance to persuasion: some contemporary approaches', in Berkowitz, L. (ed.), *Advances in Experimental Social Psychology*, Vol. 1, Academic Press, New York.
McGuire, L.W. (1985), 'Attitudes and attitude change', in Lindzey, G. and Aronson, E. (eds), *The Handbook of Social Psychology*, Vol. 2, Random House, New York.
Mullen, P.D., Green, L.W. and Persinger, G. (1985), 'Clinical trials of patient education for chronic conditions: a comparative meta-analysis of intervention types', *Preventive Medicine*, 14, pp. 753-781.
Paulussen, T. and Bartels, F. (1992), *AIDS Education for Secondary Schools and the Use of National Curricula* (in Dutch), National Centre for Health Education, Utrecht.
Petty, R.E. and Cacioppo, R.T. (1986), 'The elaboration likelihood model of persuasion', in Berkowitz, L. (ed.), *Advances in Experimental Social Psychology*, Vol. 19, Academic Press, New York.
Richard, R. and Van der Pligt, J. (1991), 'Factors affecting condom use among adolescents', *Journal of Community and Applied Social Psychology*, 1 (2), pp. 105-116.
Rogers, E.M. (1983), *Diffusion of Innovations*, The Free Press, New York.
Rogers, R.W. (1983), 'Cognitive and physiological processes in fear appeals and attitude change: a revised theory of protection motivation', in Cacioppo, J.T. and Petty, R.E. (eds), *Social Psychophysiology: A Source Book*, Guilford, New York.
Schaalma, H.P., Kok, G.J., Braeken, D., Schopman, M. and Deven, F. (1991), 'Sex and AIDS education for adolescents', *Tijdschrift voor Seksuologie*, 15, pp. 140-149.
Schaalma, H.P., Kok, G.J. and Peters, L. (1993a), 'Determinants of consistent condom use by adolescents: the impact of experience of sexual intercourse', *Health Education Research*, 8 (2), pp. 255-269.
Schaalma, H.P., Peters, L. and Kok, G.J. (1993b), 'Reactions among Dutch youth toward people with AIDS', *Journal of School Health*, April 1993, pp. 182-187.
Suls, J. and Wils, T.A. (1991), *Social Comparison*, Erlbaum, Hillsdale, NJ.
Sussman, S. (1991), 'Curriculum development in school-based prevention research', *Health Education Research*, 6 (3), pp. 339-351.
Tanner, W.M. and Pollack, R.H. (1988), 'The effect of condom use and erotic instructions on attitudes toward condoms', *Journal of Sex Research*, 25, pp. 537-541.

US Department of Health and Human Services (1984), *Methods, Examples and Resources for Improving Health Messages and Materials*, National Cancer Institute, Bethesda, Maryland.
Vogels and Van der Vliet (1990), *Youth and Sex* (in Dutch), SDU, The Hague.
Weiner B. (1986), *An Attributional Theory of Motivation and Emotion*, Springer Verlag, New York.
Weinstein, N.D. (1989), 'Effects of personal experience on self-protective behavior', *Psychological Bulletin*, 105, pp. 31-50.
Zimbardo, P.G. and Leippe, M.R. (1991), *The Psychology of Attitude Change and Social Influence*, Temple University Press, Philadelphia.

10 Demographic inputs and health outcomes: Psychological processes as mediators

D.R. Rutter and Lyn Quine

Introduction

The central issue addressed by the contributors to this book has been how do social psychological processes influence health and safety outcomes. Much of the work has made use of expectancy-value and risk perception models, and the wide variety of outcomes discussed in the chapters has shown how successful such approaches can be. Our purpose in this final chapter is to try to place social psychological research in a wider context, in which the *processes* the book has explored are seen as helping to explain the known 'epidemiological facts' about health outcomes. We shall begin by contrasting social psychological research with epidemiological research; we shall suggest a conceptual framework for combining the two traditions; we shall illustrate the approach with examples from our own research; and we shall end by considering the implications of what we have said, for theory and for empirical research.

Epidemiological and social psychological approaches to health

Epidemiological approaches

The main concern of epidemiology is to establish the incidence and prevalence of health outcomes, and to try to explain the data through what might be called 'social inputs' — principally demographic indices such as sex, age, and social class. Occasionally the outcome is a 'soft' one — attendance for screening, for example, or satisfaction with a medical intervention — but typically epidemiologists concern themselves with 'hard' outcomes, notably mortality and morbidity.

A good example of the epidemiological tradition comes from research on infant mortality. In the mid-nineteenth century more than 15 per cent of children in England and Wales died before their first birthday. At the turn of the century the figure was little changed, but then a steep decline began as rudimentary state health care and later the full National Health Service developed. By 1960 the figure was just over 2 per cent, and in 1984 it fell below 1 per cent for the first time. Infant mortality is considered to be one of the most important indices of a nation's health, but part of its special significance is what it tells us about social differentiation, *within* a nation. For example, it is well established that infant mortality is strongly linked to the social class of the parents, so much so that, even in the latest data (Figure 10.1), the ratio for Social Class V to Social Class I is 1.6:1, while the ratio for postneonatal mortality (death between 28 days and 12 months of the birth) is higher still, at 2.1:1. Postneonatal mortality is particularly important because the child who dies after the first month of life will normally have been discharged from hospital, and deficiencies in NHS neonatal care are therefore less likely to play a part than domestic social and environmental factors. Consistent with this argument, the *causes* of postneonatal mortality are distributed evenly across the classes, unlike the overall *rates*, indicating that something that may kill at the bottom of the social scale when it occurs may well not kill at the top. The implication is that working class circumstances produce a non-specific 'general vulnerability'. The theoretical question is how can that 'general vulnerability' be explained?

At first there was little attempt at explanation, but in 1980 the position changed dramatically with the publication of what was to become known as the Black Report. Black first assembled the epidemiological facts, and showed that adult mortality revealed the same pattern as infant mortality: a steadily increasing gradient from the top of the social scale to the bottom, and a gradient even *within* social classes (Marmot, Shipley and Rose, 1984; Marmot, 1986; Davey Smith, Shipley and Rose, 1990; North et al, 1993). He then proposed three possible theories as to why social inequalities occurred. The first was that the reported inequalities were artifacts of the ways in which social class, and perhaps inequalities too, were defined and measured (Illsley, 1986; LeGrand, 1985). Changes over time in the comparison of occupational groupings, in the criteria for assigning people to categories, and in the personnel making the assignments, could all lead to apparent inequalities if people who were unhealthy at Time 2 were placed in a lower category than at Time 1. The second theory was that inequalities were real rather than apparent and occurred because people who were unhealthy or potentially unhealthy were 'selected' for low status occupations or 'drifted downwards' into

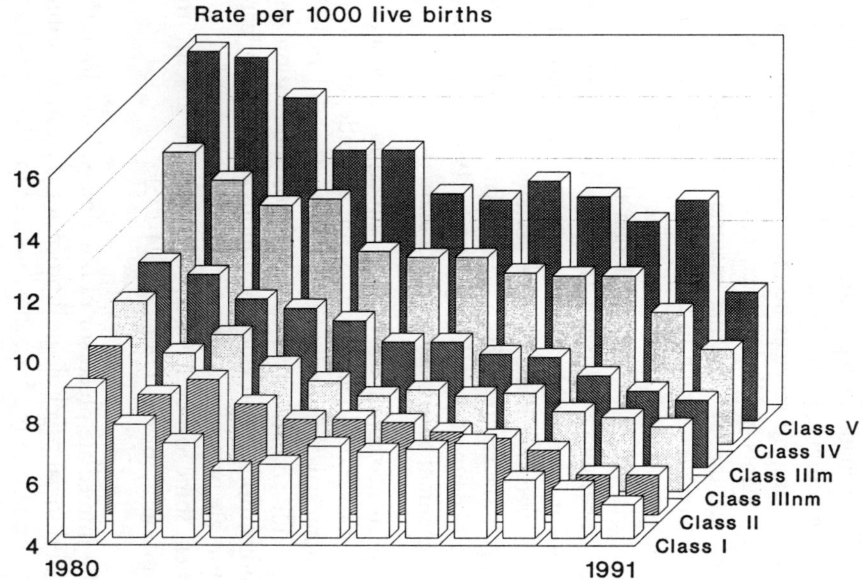

Source: OPCS Series DH3
Overall rate for 1991: 7.2

Figure 10.1 Infant mortality in England and Wales

them, while healthy people were selected or climbed upwards (Illsley, 1980, 1986; Illsley and LeGrand, 1987; LeGrand, 1986; Stern, 1983). The third theory was that people at the bottom of the social scale suffered material deprivation, which affected their health behaviours and outcomes. The 'strongest' form of the theory was structural, and said that material deprivation affected outcomes *directly*. For example, people at the bottom of the scale worked in occupations with high levels of industrial accidents, and lived in overcrowded housing which might be damp, and the individual played little if any part in mediating the effects. The second version of the theory said that material deprivation operated *indirectly*, and had its effects through the individual's behaviour. For example, lack of money prevented people taking up services because time and travel were expensive, and similar arguments applied to diet, healthy leisure, and so on. The third form of the theory was that material deprivation itself *produced* inappropriate behaviours, which in turn were responsible for the observed negative outcomes.

At the end of his analysis, Black (1980) concluded that 'it is in some form or forms of the "materialist" approach that the best answer lies' (Black, 1980, p. 120), and it is probably fair to say that the majority of subsequent writers agree (see, for example, the reviews by the British Medical Association, 1987; Macintyre, 1986, 1988; Wilkinson, 1986, 1994; Whitehead, 1987; Carroll, Bennett and Davey Smith, 1993). To quote Black again, this time on infant mortality in particular:

> to [these] basic material needs [for material resources] must be added other cognitive and motivational factors which are not independent of the distribution of material advantage. Those factors would include knowledge, certain skills and resources in verbal communication and a high level of motivation to provide continuous and loving care. When all these factors are present the infant's chance of survival is very good indeed. When some or even many of these are absent, the outlook is less propitious. (Black, 1980, pp. 124-125)

To the extent that the immediate precursor of outcome is behaviour, the role for psychological and social psychological processes is clear, according to Black: to provide the underpinning for behaviour and for the links back to social inputs. The question now becomes what *processes* do those underpinnings and links consist of. It is to processes that social psychologists have devoted most of their attention, and we now turn to this second tradition of research.

Social psychological approaches

It is useful to divide social psychological processes into two groups: socio-emotional, and cognitive. In the former we include life events, social support, and emotion, all of which have been shown to have significant effects on health outcomes (Rutter, Quine and Chesham, 1993). By way of illustration we shall consider social support.

The notion that social support might contribute to mental and physical health has its origins in a series of theories about social networks (Litwak and Szelenyi, 1969), social disorganization (Leighton, Harding, Macklin, Hughes and Leighton, 1963), and the basic human need for social transactions (Maslow, 1968). In the mid 1970s three major papers were published which reviewed the mounting evidence (Cassel, 1976; Cobb, 1976; Kaplan, Cassel and Gore, 1977). Protective effects of social support were demonstrated for numerous disease outcomes, including overall mortality, pregnancy outcome, psychiatric illness, suicide, accidents, recovery from illness, and death from chronic disease (Broadhead et al., 1983). Since those papers there has been a huge body of research on the relationship of social support to both physical and psychiatric morbidity (for reviews see Mueller, 1980; Greenblatt, Becerra and Serafetinides, 1982; Thoits, 1982; Broadhead et al., 1983; Monroe, 1983; Schradle and Dougher, 1985; Alloway and Bebbington, 1987), and several hypotheses have emerged. The original hypothesis was that social support provided a buffer against adversity but had no independent effect in the absence of adversity (Dean and Lin, 1977). However, research by Henderson et al. (1978a and b) suggested that it might have both direct and independent effects on mental and/or physical health regardless of whether adversity was experienced. A third version of the theory argued that social support has a therapeutic effect after the onset of a particular disorder, shortening the episode and reducing symptoms. Lastly it has been suggested that social support could be deleterious for some members of the community, particularly elderly people (Lowenthal, 1964).

The evidence for a relationship between social support and *physical* health has been reviewed by Berkman (1984, 1986). Berkman argues that there is increasing evidence from prospective epidemiological investigations that social support reduces mortality. The relationship is stronger for men than women, but the mechanisms by which social support has its effects are poorly understood. Berkman suggests that a shorter life and poor social relationships may both be related to personality traits, of which neuroticism and anxiety are among the most important.

In *mental* health, there is again relatively little prospective data, but a plethora of cross-sectional studies has been published showing a relationship with social support (Cohen and Sokolovsky, 1978; Henderson et al., 1978a and b). However, the evidence is open to a number of interpretations, as we have hinted already. One is that poor social support causes mental ill-health, while another is that people who are depressed withdraw socially, or simply have a gloomy view of their social networks. Of the prospective studies, some have tested for buffering and some for an independent effect, but the findings have been equivocal (Henderson et al., 1981; Pearlin, Lieberman, Menaghan and Mullan, 1981; Lin and Dean, 1984; Brown et al., 1986a and b). Henderson's study, for example, found an association between reported inadequacy of social support and the onset of symptoms of neurotic illness in the presence of life events, but a measure of neuroticism accounted for much more of the variance in subsequent symptoms (69 per cent). Brown's ambitious study, on the other hand, based on a sample of 395 working class women, found that for married women the existence of a confiding relationship measured at Time 1 was not associated with a lower risk of depression in the succeeding year; but, in contrast, single mothers were less likely to become depressed if they did have access to socially supportive relationships. To try to resolve the differences between the two approaches, Henderson and Brown subsequently worked together, to produce a critical review (Henderson and Brown, 1988), and not surprisingly the main emphasis of the paper was methodological.

As we saw earlier, Henderson has argued that the best way to disentangle cause and effect is to mount intervention studies, in which social support is manipulated systematically. Impressive evidence has come recently from intervention studies in pregnancy (Klaus, Kennell, Robertson and Sosa, 1986; Flint and Poulengeris, 1987; Oakley, 1988; Elbourne and Oakley, 1990). In the most recent of the studies, by Oakley, Rajan and Grant (1990), 509 women with a history of low birthweight took part. Half received extra social support in addition to standard antenatal care, and half did not. The extra support was given by four research midwives, who offered twenty-four hour telephone contact and a programme of home visits. Babies in the intervention group had a mean birthweight 38g higher than the babies in the control group, and there were fewer very low birthweight babies. More women in the control group were admitted to hospital during pregnancy, while spontaneous onset of labour and spontaneous vaginal delivery were more common in the intervention group, who also required less epidural anaesthesia. Babies in the intervention group required less intensive care and special neonatal care, and were significantly healthier in the early weeks, as were their mothers. There could be little doubt that the effects had been caused by the manipulation, and social support was thus shown to be a powerful variable.

Socio-emotional processes, we suggested, are the first set of processes that social psychologists have examined. The second are cognitive processes, and a good example this time is the expectancy-value tradition in attitude research, which a number of the preceding chapters have examined. The model used most frequently in research on health has been the Health Belief Model, and an enormous amount has been published. Since the major review by Janz and Becker (1984), there have been studies on, for example, AIDS prevention (reviewed by Hayes, 1991); self-examination for breast cancer (for example Ronis and Harel, 1989; Champion, 1990); attendance for dental checks (for example Chen and Land, 1986, 1990); attendance for cervical smears (for example Hennig and Knowles, 1990); and attendance for routine medical checks (for example Norman and Fitter, 1991). The largest category, as the examples suggest, continues to be research on *preventive* health behaviours and, in general, the strongest support for the model has come from prospective studies, in which behaviour is measured some time *after* the measurement of beliefs. The leading predictor of behaviour has most commonly been perceived barriers, which means that the most likely people to take up the preventive behaviour are those who see the costs as minimal. Perceived susceptibility is often a stronger predictor than perceived benefits — even though most people apparently see themselves as relatively invulnerable to almost all diseases, the condition known as 'unrealistic optimism' (Weinstein, 1980, 1982; Van der Pligt, this volume; Hoorens, this volume). The weakest predictor of behaviour in the Health Belief Model has generally been perceived severity, probably because people are relatively unthreatened by negative long term outcomes that are unlikely to happen and are difficult to imagine.

The other main expectancy-value approach has been the Theory of Reasoned Action, and again there is a considerable literature, much of it reviewed by Ajzen and Fishbein (1980), Canary and Siebold (1984), Sheppard, Hartwick and Warshaw (1988), Ajzen (1988, 1991), and Tesser and Shaffer (1990). Three main conclusions emerge: first, attitudes predict behaviour, and a large proportion of the variance is often explained; second, personal beliefs and attitude are generally better predictors than normative beliefs and subjective norm; and third, behaviour is predicted less well by attitudes to objects than by attitudes to related behaviours. There is, however, one important limitation to the model, namely that it applies only to behaviour that is perceived to be under the individual's control. If, for example, I have a positive attitude towards attending a clinic for a new screening service, but I cannot read the appointment card or I have no means of transport, the model will apparently *fail* to predict my intentions and behaviour. What was missing was an estimate of what Bandura called self-efficacy – 'the conviction that one can execute the behaviour required to produce the outcomes' (Bandura, 1977) – and it was that omission that the Theory of Planned Behaviour overcame (Ajzen, 1988). The theory has already been used on a variety of health behaviours – including, for example, weight loss (Schifter and Ajzen, 1985); taking exercise after giving birth (Godin, Vezina and Leclerc, 1989); limiting infants' sugar intake (Beale and Manstead, 1991); and screening, food choice, using condoms, drink-driving, and wearing cycle helmets (all in this volume) – and there is good evidence that perceived behavioural control indeed does predict intention. Whether there is also a *direct* path to behaviour, however, remains uncertain.

An integrated conceptual framework

We began the chapter by examining epidemiological approaches. Epidemiology establishes links between inputs and outcomes, but can say little about the causal mechanisms between them – the processes that explain *how* and *why* inputs lead to outcomes. We next discussed psychological and social psychological approaches, which *do* link processes to outcomes but can say little about the role of inputs. We now present an approach that attempts to combine the two traditions. It was first outlined in a review paper on pregnancy outcome (Rutter and Quine, 1990), and it was presented in detail in our book (Rutter, Quine and Chesham, 1993).

Our central argument is that social psychological processes are most usefully seen as *mediators* between social inputs and health outcomes, as the means *by which* inputs influence outcomes (Figure 10.2). We distinguish between socio-emotional and cognitive mediators, as we have made clear already, and socio-emotional variables are shown in the upper branch of the model and cognitive variables in the lower branch. *Socio-emotional* variables include people's experience of severe life events and difficulties, and the availability and adequacy of supportive relationships offering cognitive guidance, tangible assistance, emotional support, social reinforcement, and opportunities for socializing. Severe life events, in combination with low social support, we argue, will lead to emotional problems, including loss of self-esteem, anxiety, and depression. *Cognitive* variables include people's access to information and knowledge, and their

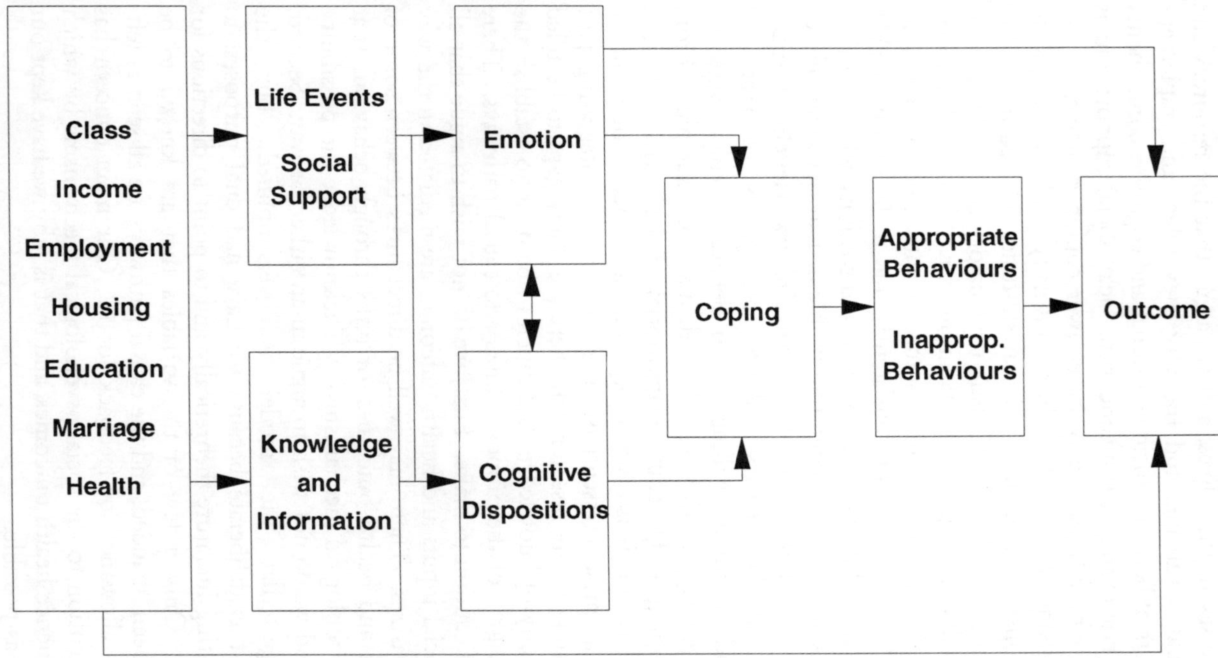

Source: Rutter, Quine and Chesham (1993)

Figure 10.2 A model of mediators in health

cognitive dispositions — by which we mean such things as perceived personal control and beliefs and attitudes, both of which we see as products of information, knowledge and communication.

At the core of our model lies coping. Coping is to do with how people confront the stresses in their lives, and we argue that the resources and strategies they have available, and the way they select and implement them, are products of both the socio-emotional and cognitive components of our model. For example, someone who lacks social support and is already weakened by adversity may have fewer coping strategies to call upon than someone who is free from adversity and has access to supportive relationships, and the particular strategies selected may differ too. Again, someone with an optimistic explanatory style, who focuses on external, unstable, and specific explanations for life's difficulties, may display different coping patterns from someone with a pessimistic style, who expects bad events to occur consistently and to be uncontrollable, and who reacts with helplessness, depression, and passivity whenever they do occur. Socio-emotional and cognitive problems may act separately or in combination, and will result in coping styles and strategies characterized by helplessness or hopelessness, altered perceptions of risk and vulnerability, and an undue willingness to behave in risky ways, by smoking in pregnancy or driving when drunk, for example. From dysfunctional coping styles come inappropriate behaviours, and from inappropriate behaviours it is a small step to negative health outcomes.

Our model is at present essentially a framework for integrating past findings and guiding future research, for there are many gaps to be filled in the existing body of knowledge, and much to be done to establish the strengths and weights of the proposed links and causal pathways. There are two points of caution to make. First, we do not wish to argue that all links between social inputs and health outcomes are mediated in the way the model emphasizes. There may well be direct links between some of the social inputs and health outcomes, or links through behaviour that bypass social psychological mechanisms. We acknowledge the possibility of other links, and we do not wish to argue in an either/or way. Second, we acknowledge that the model is oversimplified, but the oversimplification is deliberate because we have had dual purposes: to integrate the existing literature theoretically and to point to directions for future research. Only a few of the variables that are known to be important have been included, and the causal pathways are all seen as left-to-right with no allowance for feedback loops. Our main concern has been to draw attention to the social psychological mechanisms by which social inputs influence health outcomes, and that is why we have kept our model as simple as possible.

A useful example to illustrate the workings of the model is provided by the link we have discussed already between social class and pregnancy outcome. It is well established that, the further down the social scale one goes, the greater the incidence of low birthweight — just as with infant mortality. The question of course is why and, by integrating the known facts, our model can help to provide an answer. First, it is known that more working class women than middle class women smoke during pregnancy (Oakley, 1989), and it is established that smoking leads to low birthweight (Froggatt, 1988). There are also suggestions in the literature that smoking in young mothers is an attempt to cope with stress (Graham, 1976, 1984), and that stress often arises from severe negative life events that have to be faced in the absence of social support (Brown and Harris, 1978; Oakley, Rajan and Grant, 1990). The evidence suggests furthermore that working class women have a more positive attitude than middle class women to smoking (Marsh and Matheson, 1983) — perhaps through poor education or limited access to information. Thus, we suggest, the material deprivation experienced by working class women leads first to severe life events and lack of social support, and to poor education and access to information. The former leads on to negative emotions, and the latter to negative attitudes and dispositions. The socio-emotional and cognitive factors combine into poor coping, which in turn is reflected in inappropriate behaviours such as smoking. Smoking leads finally to poor outcome.

As we have acknowledged, our model is a deliberately oversimplified account of what are complex issues, and the outline we have given in our example is oversimplified too. Nevertheless, it serves to illustrate the way in which two apparently disparate traditions can be combined, we hope profitably, and it points to hypotheses that can be tested empirically. As to how the model can be tested, we turn now to examples from our own research. We shall examine three in particular: the effects of social class on mothers' satisfaction with maternity care; the influence of education and social class on women's responses to breast cancer screening; and the association between age and motorcycling safety.

A programme of research

Social class and mothers' satisfaction with maternity care

Our first study was published by Quine, Rutter and Gowen (1993). Sixty first-time mothers-to-be were approached towards the end of their pregnancies during maternity classes organized by a local hospital. Our objective was to examine the effects of social class on satisfaction with maternity care, and to explore the possibility that a number of social psychological mediators might also play a part: the woman's knowledge and information about pregnancy and childbirth; how prepared she felt for the birth; how much support she felt she had from her family and friends; and how much pain she expected and subsequently experienced. The design of the study was prospective: information, preparation, support, and expected pain were measured by means of a questionnaire completed when the women were first approached at the classes; and retrospective measures of preparation, support, and actual pain were collected by interviewing the women at home shortly after the birth. A rating of overall satisfaction with the quality of the birth experience was also taken during the follow-up home visit.

Our analyses used path analysis, and the results are shown in Figure 10.3. The total variance explained was 53 per cent, and social class affected both social support and information at Time 1: working class women felt less supported than middle class women, and they felt less informed. Women who felt supported at Time 1 reported less pain during the birth than those who felt they were not receiving adequate support, and women who felt less pain in turn reported greater satisfaction with the birth experience. Women who felt informed felt more prepared for the birth, and preparation also led to greater satisfaction with the birth experience.

The results offer good support for our model, for they demonstrate the importance of both social support and adequate information as *mediators* between social class and the experience of childbirth. Working class women appear to be disadvantaged in both respects: they are less supported than middle class women, and they lack adequate information. They are consequently less likely to find childbirth a rewarding experience. In line with our *descriptive* findings, *intervention* studies in which women are offered social support during pregnancy and labour typically find that support has positive effects (Sosa et al., 1980; Oakley, 1985; Oakley and Rajan, 1991) — fewer admissions to hospital during pregnancy, shorter labours, greater awareness during delivery, less use of neonatal intensive care by babies, greater health service use by mothers and babies after the birth, greater satisfaction with care, and improved psychological well-being, especially reduced anxiety. Women who also feel they have adequate information are more likely to feel prepared for the birth and so are more satisfied with the experience. Social class does not have a *direct* effect on outcome, however; instead, it operates through social support on the one hand and information on the other.

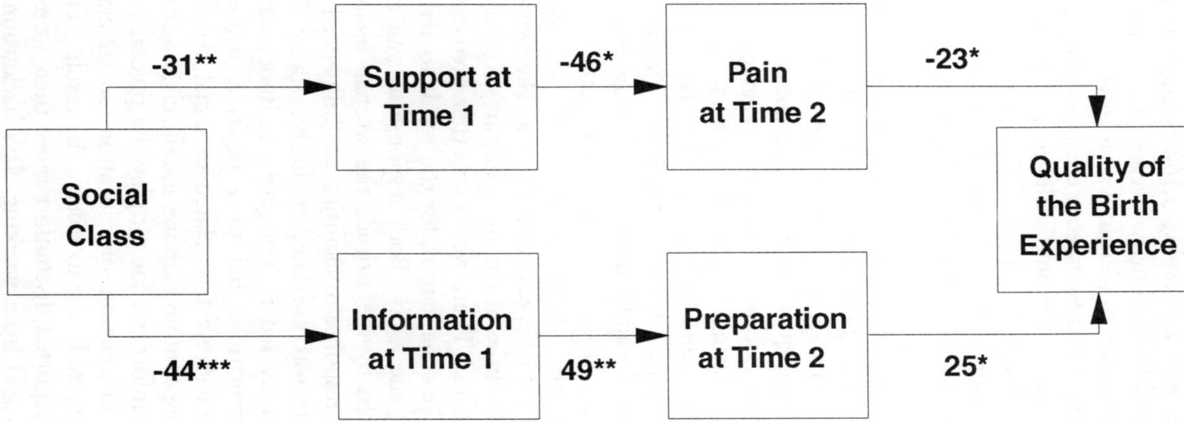

Variance explained 53%.
*p<0.05 **p<0.01 ***p<0.001
Source: Quine, Rutter and Gowen (1993)

Figure 10.3 Quality of the birth experience

Our second study was published by Vaile, Calnan, Rutter and Wall (1993). Once again the design was prospective and longitudinal. Shortly before they were to be invited for X-ray mammography, 3,160 women in the South-East Thames Regional Health Authority were sent a postal questionnaire. Its objectives were twofold: to identify variables that would predict attendance and nonattendance; and to explore the possibility that characteristics of respondents at Time 1 would help to explain their responses at Time 2. The questionnaire included items about the woman's education and social class, her experience of previous screening visits and clinical breast examinations, if any, and her attitude and subjective norm about being screened.

After screening had taken place, the women were followed up. Those who had completed the first postal questionnaire, had attended for screening, and had received a negative result (that is, no evidence of abnormality) were sent a second postal questionnaire. The questionnaire asked what had made the woman decide to be screened, what practical difficulties if any she had had in getting to the clinic, what she had thought of the staff and facilities there, and how she had felt about the X-ray itself, including whether it had caused discomfort or pain. Finally, we asked about satisfaction with the service and whether the woman thought she would return in three years' time when she was invited again.

Our main results are shown in a path diagram (Figure 10.4). The most important predictors of satisfaction, it emerged, were the way the woman responded to the staff and to the facilities at the unit, in part, no doubt, a reflection of objective characteristics. There were two other predictors, however, both of them negative: the time it took for the result to arrive, and discomfort experienced during the X-ray. Both response to staff and response to facilities were influenced by the attitude the woman *brought to* her screening appointment, and response to facilities was influenced by subjective norm as well. Attitude was unrelated to health status, but previous experience of mammography led to a negative attitude, while experience of other clinical examinations led to a positive attitude. Experience of clinical breast examinations was related to social class, in that clinical examinations were more common among middle class women than working class women. Discomfort, we found, played a pivotal role, for it mediated the effects upon satisfaction of education, social class, previous clinical breast examination, and time to receive the result. That is, educated, middle class women reported discomfort more than women without educational qualifications and from working class backgrounds, and discomfort was greatest in women who had had clinical breast

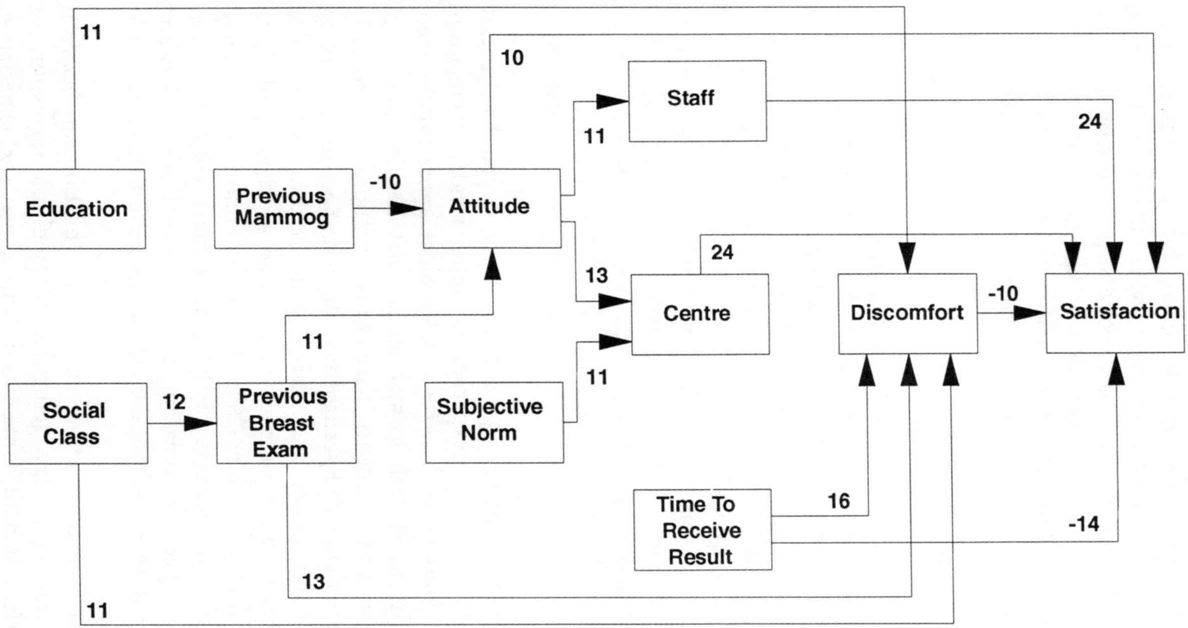

Variance explained 28.6%
All beta weights $p<0.001$
Source: Vaile, Calnan, Rutter and Wall (1993)

Figure 10.4 Satisfaction with breast cancer screening

examinations before and who had had to wait a long time for their present result to arrive.

As in the study of pregnancy outcome, our model received good support. The strongest predictors of satisfaction were the woman's perceptions of the staff and centre where she was screened, but perceptions were underpinned by attitude, which in turn was influenced by class. Moreover, both class and education had direct effects on discomfort, the other outcome measure, which was also a significant predictor of satisfaction. There were thus both direct and indirect paths from social inputs to outcome, and social psychological processes acted as mediators.

Age and motorcycling safety

Our third and final study was published in Rutter, Quine and Chesham (1993). Once again, the design was prospective and longitudinal. From a national sample of registered motorcycle keepers, 2,050 were sent a postal questionnaire designed to tap their beliefs and attitudes about safe riding, their self-reported behaviours and accidents during the previous year, and their demographic characteristics. A year later, a second questionnaire was posted, this time asking about behaviour and accidents since the first questionnaire. It is well established that young male riders aged twenty-four or under have a higher accident rate than any other group of motorcyclists (Department of Transport, 1993), and our objective was to examine the possibility that behaviour and attitudes were mediators.

In the twelve months to Time 2, 13.6 per cent of the sample had at least one spill or accident. Young, inexperienced, trained riders were more likely to report accidents than those who were older, more experienced, and untrained, while riders with formal educational qualifications were more likely to have had accidents than those without — probably reflecting age and experience and perhaps training too. Speeding, breaking traffic laws, riding too close, and losing concentration all revealed significant differences between riders who reported accidents and those who did not, and the differences held for both Time 1 and Time 2 behaviour. Principal components analysis at Time 1 confirmed that breaking traffic laws, speeding, breaking the Highway Code, and riding too close belonged together, and we named the factor Breaking Law and Rules.

The next stage of our analysis was to examine the relationship between social inputs and breaking the law and rules. By multiple regression we were able to show that, at both Time 1 and Time 2, age, sex, experience, and formal training were all significant predictors, and the relationships were similar on the two occasions. The most likely riders to report violations were those who were young, male, inexperienced, and formally trained. Age was much the strongest predictor, but all the variables taken together accounted for around a quarter of the variance. Principal components analysis of the attitude data at Time 1 revealed four behavioural belief factors and two normative belief factors, and just two factors predicted violations: attitude to breaking law and rules, and attitude to taking care. By means of path analysis, finally, we were able to show that both age and sex led directly to behaviour (Figure 10.5), but were also mediated – age by attitude to obeying the law and rules of safe riding (negatively), sex by attitude to taking care (positively, perhaps through 'risk compensation'). Education also led indirectly to behaviour, again through attitude to taking care.

Once again there was good evidence for our model. Behaviour was predicted by social inputs, notably age and education, and attitudes acted as mediators, though there were also strong direct paths from inputs to behaviour. The evidence thus suggests that demography has at least some of its effects on behaviour 'through' attitudes, so that an important part of being a young rider is the attitudes that youth brings with it. The indication is that social psychological variables have a significant part to play in a theoretical account of accident involvement, and that our model offers a useful framework.

Conclusion: theoretical and empirical implications of the model

The main tenet of our chapter has been that social psychological variables are best seen as mediators between social inputs and health outcomes. We have seen our task as twofold: to explore which variables are important for which areas of health; and to draw out the possible links. The question we address finally is what does our approach offer that traditional approaches do not – where traditional approaches confine themselves to epidemiology or to social psychology, but pay little attention to the links between them.

There are three main answers. First, through our model we are able to posit at least some of the mechanisms and processes that 'explain' the facts that epidemiology has revealed. For example, infant mortality is greater in working class families than in middle class families, and we have been able to suggest at least part of the answer to the question why: the link is *mediated*, through life events, social support, cognitive dispositions, coping, and behaviour. Again, as we have seen, young male motorcyclists have higher accident rates than other motorcyclists, and again mediation helps

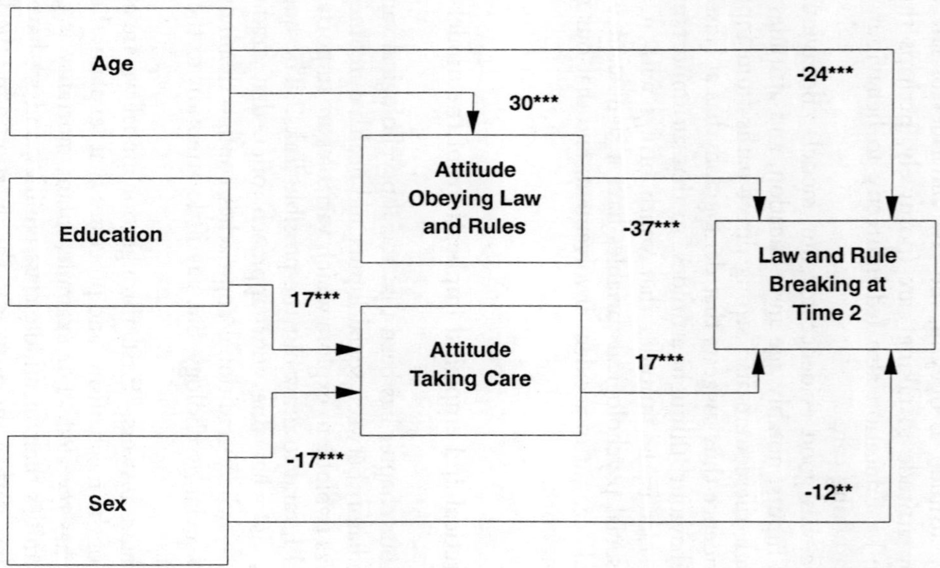

Variance explained 31%
**p<0.01 ***p<0.001
Source: Rutter, Quine and Chesham (1993)

Figure 10.5 Motorcycling safety

to explain the relationship: this time, locus of control, cognitive dispositions, and behaviour are the most important social psychological variables.

The second answer is that our approach is able to *quantify* the patterns of mediation, by means of path analysis. That is, we are able to *weight* the relative importance of the mediating variables and to test their strengths statistically. The third answer, which leads on from the second, is that we are able to test when effects are direct and when they are indirect. For example, we knew from the literature that middle class women are generally less satisfied than working class women with breast screening, but we did not know whether the path was direct or indirect. By using the framework provided by our model we were able to show that it was indirect, through discomfort: middle class women experienced more discomfort than working class women, and it was discomfort that made them less satisfied. For epidemiology our approach is thus able to 'explain' some of the bald epidemiological facts; and for social psychology, it puts familiar mechanisms into an epidemiological context and gives them a central role in explaining health outcomes, a role that without the links back to epidemiological social inputs they would be denied.

The remaining issues concern the future, and there are two main questions to address. The first is about the best strategy to adopt for testing the model, whether 'micro' or 'macro'. The micro or 'bottom up' approach to mediation takes one set of variables at a time — input, mediator, and outcome — and attempts to join them later. The macro or 'top down' approach offers a putative model of all the mechanisms of interest and attempts to test all the relationships at once. For practical reasons the micro approach is easier, of course, and has generally been preferred. Thus, for example, there are enormous literatures on the roles of locus of control, coping, and behaviour in mediating class and health, but because of the micro approach the literatures are more than enormous: they are separate. The time has therefore come, we believe, for a move towards macro strategies, for it is the *overall* pattern of relationships that matters most. Only through top down analyses will it be possible to determine the causal ordering of variables, their relative weights (both individually and in groups), and whether genuine mediation can be demonstrated.

This last issue, testing for the occurrence of genuine mediation, is particularly important. Although conceptually the causal pathways we have suggested may make sense, many have yet to be confirmed statistically. As Baron and Kenny (1986) point out, mediation is best tested by conducting three regression analyses: first, the mediator is regressed on the independent variable; second, the dependent variable is regressed on the independent variable; and third, the dependent variable is regressed on both the independent variable and the mediator. If mediation *is* present, three conditions will hold: the independent variable will affect the mediator in the first analysis; the independent variable will affect the dependent variable in the second analysis; and the mediator will affect the dependent variable in the third analysis. If all three conditions hold in the predicted direction, the effect of the independent variable on the dependent variable must be less in the third analysis than in the second. Full analyses of the sort that Baron and Kenny suggest have seldom been conducted as yet, and they will need extensive data collection and the continued application of sophisticated techniques of multivariate statistical analysis.

The other main issue for the future of our model concerns its limitations. The model we have outlined is intended as a framework for integrating past findings and for guiding future research. As we have said already, we do not wish to suggest that all links between social inputs and health outcomes are mediated in the way the model emphasizes. Moreover, we have acknowledged that the model is oversimplified, not least in that all the causal pathways we include are seen as left to right with no allowance for feedback loops. In fact, feedback loops are likely to be of great importance. It may be, for example, that reducing how much one smokes affects not only health outcomes but also variables that occur earlier in the model, such as perceived locus of control and attitudes. Changes in those variables may in turn encourage a further reduction in smoking, so that outcomes are improved still more. To take another example, improved coping may feed back to social support, so that people who begin to cope better make new friends, which helps them to cope better still. To establish the role of feedback, and to test the utility of the model as a whole, detailed descriptive data and controlled experimental intervention will both be necessary. As always, the first essential will be to design the research properly, in such a way that answers can be found. That is perhaps the most important message of all to come from this book.

References

Ajzen, I. (1988), *Attitudes, Personality, and Behavior*, Dorsey Press, Chicago.

Ajzen, I. (1991), 'The Theory of Planned Behavior', *Organizational Behavior and Human Decision Processes*, 50, pp. 179-211.

Ajzen, I. and Fishbein, M. (1980), *Understanding Attitudes and Predicting Social Behavior*, Prentice-Hall, Englewood Cliffs, NJ.

Alloway, R. and Bebbington, P. (1987), 'The buffer theory of social support — a review of the literature', *Psychological Medicine*, 17, pp. 91-108.
Bandura, A. (1977), 'Self-efficacy: toward a unifying theory of behavioral change', *Psychological Review*, 84, pp. 191-215.
Baron, R.M. and Kenny, D.A. (1986), 'The moderator-mediator variable distinction in social psychological research: conceptual, strategic, and statistical considerations', *Journal of Personality and Social Psychology*, 51, pp. 1173-82.
Beale, D.A. and Manstead, A.S.R. (1991), 'Predicting mothers' intentions to limit frequency of infants' sugar intake: testing the theory of planned behavior', *Journal of Applied Social Psychology*, 21, pp. 409-431.
Berkman, L.F. (1984), 'Assessing the physical health effects of social networks and support', *Review of Public Health*, 5, pp. 413-432.
Berkman, L.F. (1986), 'Social networks, support and health: taking the next step forward', *American Journal of Epidemiology*, 123, pp. 559-162.
Black, D. (1980), *Inequalities in Health* (Black Report), Report of a research working group chaired by Sir Douglas Black, London, DHSS.
BMA (1987), *Deprivation and Ill Health*, Board of Science and Education, British Medical Association.
Broadhead, W.E., Kaplan, B.H., Sherman, A.J., Wagner, E.H., Schoenback, V.J., Grimson, R., Heyden, S., Tibblin, G. and Gehlbach, S.H. (1983), 'The epidemiologic evidence for a relationship between social support and health', *American Journal of Epidemiology*, 117, pp. 521-537.
Brown, G.W., Andrews, B., Harris, T., Adler, Z. and Bridge, L. (1986a), 'Social support, self-esteem and depression', *Psychological Medicine*, 16, pp. 813-31.
Brown, G.W., Bifulco, A., Harris, T. and Bridge, L. (1986b), 'Life stress, chronic subclinical symptoms and vulnerability to clinical depression', *Journal of Affective Disorders*, 11, pp. 1-9.
Brown, G.W. and Harris, T. (1978), *Social Origins of Depression: A Study of Psychiatric Disorder in Women*, Tavistock, London.
Canary, D.J. and Siebold, D.R. (1984), *Attitudes and Behavior: An Annotated Bibliography*, Praeger, New York.
Carroll, D., Bennett, P. and Davey Smith, G. (1993), 'Socio-economic health inequalities: their origins and implications', *Psychology and Health*, 8, pp. 295-316.
Cassel, J. (1976), 'The contribution of the social environment to host resistance', *American Journal of Epidemiology*, 104, pp. 107-23.
Champion, V.L. (1990), 'Breast self-examination in women 35 and older: a prospective study', *Journal of Behavioral Medicine*, 13, pp. 523-538.

Chen, M. and Land, K.C. (1986), 'Testing the Health Belief Model: LISREL analysis of alternative models of causal relationships between health beliefs and preventive dental behavior', *Social Psychology Quarterly*, 49, pp. 56-60.

Chen, M. and Land, K.C. (1990), 'Socioeconomic status (SES) and the Health Belief Model: LISREL analysis of unidimensional versus multidimensional formulations', *Journal of Social Behavior and Personality*, 5, pp. 263-284.

Cobb, S. (1976), 'Social support as a moderator of life stress', *Psychosomatic Medicine*, 38, pp. 300-314.

Cohen, C. and Sokolovsky, J. (1978), 'Schizophrenia and social networks', *Schizophrenia Bulletin*, 4, pp. 546-560.

Davey Smith, G., Shipley, M.J. and Rose, G. (1990), 'Magnitude and causes of socioeconomic differentials in mortality: further evidence from the Whitehall Study', *Journal of Epidemiology and Community Health*, 44, pp. 265-270.

Dean, A. and Lin, N. (1977), 'The stress-buffering role of social support: problems and prospects for systematic investigation', *Journal of Nervous and Mental Disease*, 165, 6, pp. 403-17.

Department of Transport (1993) *Road Accidents Great Britain 1992: The Casualty Report*. London: HMSO.

Elbourne, D. and Oakley, A. (1990), 'An overview of trials of social support during pregnancy: effects on gestational age at delivery and birthweight', in Berendes, H.W., Kessel, W. and Yaffe, S. (eds), *Advances in the Prevention of Low Birthweight*, Perinatology Press, New York.

Flint, C. and Poulengeris, P. (1987), *Know Your Midwife*, Heinemann, London.

Froggatt, P. (1988), *Fourth Report of the Independent Scientific Committee on Smoking and Health*, HMSO, London.

Godin, G., Vezina, L. and Leclerc, O. (1989), 'Factors influencing intentions of pregnant women to exercise after giving birth', *Public Health Reports*, 104, pp. 188-195.

Graham, H. (1976), 'Smoking in pregnancy: the attitudes of expectant mothers', *Social Science and Medicine*, 10, pp. 399-405.

Graham, H. (1984), *Women, Health and the Family*, Wheatsheaf, Brighton.

Greenblatt, M., Becerra, R.M. and Serafetinides, E.A. (1982), 'Social networks and mental health: an overview', *American Journal of Psychiatry*, 139, 8, pp. 977-84.

Hayes, J.A. (1991), 'Psychological barriers to behavior change in preventing human immunodeficiency virus (HIV) infection', *Counselling Psychologist*, 19, pp. 585-602.

Henderson, A.S. and Brown, G.W. (1988), 'Social support: the hypothesis and the evidence', in Henderson, A.S. and Burrows, G.D. (eds), *Handbook of Social Psychiatry*, Elsevier, Amsterdam.

Henderson, A.S., Byrne, D.G. and Duncan-Jones, P. (1981), *Neurosis and the Social Environment*, Academic Press, Sydney.

Henderson, A.S., Byrne, D.G., Duncan-Jones, P., Adcock, S., Scott, R. and Steele, G.P. (1978a), 'Social bonds in the epidemiology of neurosis: a preliminary communication', *British Journal of Psychiatry*, 132, pp. 463-466.

Henderson, A.S., Duncan-Jones, P., McAuley, H. and Ritchie, K. (1978b), 'The patient's primary group', *British Journal of Psychiatry*, 132, pp. 74-86.

Hennig, P. and Knowles, A. (1990), 'Factors influencing women over 40 years to take precautions against cervical cancer', *Journal of Applied Social Psychology*, 20, pp. 1612-1621.

Illsley, R. (1980), *Professional or Public Health: Sociology in Health and Medicine*, London, Nuffield Provincial Hospitals Trust.

Illsley, R. (1986), 'Occupational class, selection and the production of inequalities in health', *Quarterly Journal of Social Affairs*, 2, pp. 151-165.

Illsley, R. and LeGrand, J. (1987), 'The measurement of inequality', LSE Welfare State Programme Discussion Paper No. 12, London, LSE.

Janz, N.K. and Becker, M.H. (1984), 'The Health Belief Model: a decade later', *Health Education Quarterly*, 11, pp. 1-47.

Kaplan, B.H., Cassel, J.C. and Gore, S. (1977), 'Social support and health', *Medical Care*, 15, 5, Suppl., pp. 47-58.

Klaus, M.H., Kennell, J.H., Robertson, S.S. and Sosa, R. (1986), 'Effects of social support during parturition on maternal and infant morbidity', *British Medical Journal*, 293, pp. 585-7.

LeGrand, J. (1985), 'Inequalities in health: the human capital approach', LSE Welfare State Programme Discussion Paper No. 1, LSE, London.

LeGrand, J. (1986), 'Inequalities in health and health care: a research agenda', in Wilkinson, R.G. (ed.), *Class and Health*, London, Tavistock, pp. 115-125.

Leighton, D.C., Harding, J.S., Macklin, D.B., Hughes, C.C. and Leighton, A.H. (1963), 'Psychiatric findings of the Stirling County Study', *American Journal of Psychiatry*, 119, pp. 1021-6.

Lin, N. and Dean, A. (1984), 'Social support and depression: a panel study', *Social Psychiatry*, 19, pp. 83-91.

Litwak, E. and Szelenyi, I. (1969), 'Primary group structures and their functions: kin, neighbors and friends', *American Sociological Review*, 34, pp. 465-481.

Lowenthal, M.F. (1964), 'Social isolation and mental illness in old age', *American Sociological Review*, 29, pp. 54-70.
Macintyre, S. (1986), 'The patterning of health by social position in contemporary Britain: directions for sociological research', *Social Science and Medicine*, 23, pp. 393-415.
Macintyre, S. (1988), 'A review of the social patterning and significance of measures of height, weight, blood pressure and respiratory function', *Social Science and Medicine*, 27, pp. 327-337.
Marmot, M.G. (1986), 'Social inequalities in mortality: the social environment', in Wilkinson R.G. (ed.), *Class and Health*, London and New York, Tavistock.
Marmot, M.G., Shipley, M.J. and Rose, G. (1984), 'Inequalities in death — specific explanations of a general pattern?', *The Lancet*, May 5, 1984, pp. 1003-1006.
Marsh, A. and Matheson, J. (1983), *Smoking Attitudes and Behaviour*, OPCS Report SS1153, HMSO, London.
Maslow, A.H. (1968), *Toward a Psychology of Being*, Van Nostrand, New York.
Monroe, S.M. (1983), 'Social support and disorder: toward an untangling of cause and effect', *American Journal of Community Psychology*, 11, 1, pp. 81-97.
Mueller, D.P. (1980), 'Social networks: a promising direction for research on the relationship of the social environment to psychiatric disorder', *Social Science and Medicine*, 14, pp. 147-161.
Norman, P. and Fitter, M. (1991), 'Predicting attendance at health screening: organisational factors and patients' health beliefs', *Counselling Psychology Quarterly*, 4, pp. 143-155.
North, F., Syme, S.L., Feeney, A., Head, J., Shipley, M.J. and Marmot, M.G. (1993), 'Explaining socioeconomic differences in sickness absence: the Whitehall II study', *British Medical Journal*, 306, pp. 361-366.
Oakley, A. (1985), 'Social support in pregnancy: the "soft" way to increase birthweight?', *Social Science and Medicine*, 21, pp. 1259-1268.
Oakley, A. (1988), 'Is social support good for the health of mothers and babies?', *Journal of Infant and Reproductive Psychology*, 6, pp. 3-21.
Oakley, A. (1989), 'Smoking in pregnancy: smokescreen or risk factor? Towards a materialist analysis', *Sociology of Health and Illness*, 11, pp. 311-335.
Oakley, A. and Rajan, L. (1991), 'Social class and social support: the same or different?', *Sociology*, 25, pp. 31-59.
Oakley, A., Rajan, L. and Grant, A. (1990), 'Social support and pregnancy outcome', *British Journal of Obstetrics and Gynaecology*, 97, pp. 155-162.

Pearlin, L.I., Lieberman, M.A., Menaghan, E.G. and Mullan, J.P. (1981), 'The stress process', *Journal of Health and Social Behavior*, 22, pp. 337-356.
Quine, L., Rutter, D.R. and Gowen, S. (1993), 'Women's satisfaction with the quality of the birth experience: a prospective study of social and psychological predictors', *Journal of Infant and Reproductive Psychology*, 11, pp. 107-113.
D.L. and Harel, Y. (1989), 'Health beliefs and breast examination behaviors: analyses of linear structural relations', *Psychology and Health*, 3, pp. 259-285.
Rutter, D.R. and Quine, L. (1990), 'Inequalities in pregnancy outcome: a review of psychosocial and behavioural mediators', *Social Science and Medicine*, 30, pp. 553-568.
Rutter, D.R., Quine, L. and Chesham, D.J., (1993), *Social Psychological Approaches to Health*, Harvester Wheatsheaf, Hemel Hempstead.
Schifter, D.B. and Ajzen, I. (1985), 'Intention, perceived control, and weight loss: an application of the theory of planned behavior', *Journal of Personality and Social Psychology*, 49, pp. 843-851.
Schradle, S.B. and Dougher, M.J. (1985), 'Social support as a mediator of stress: theoretical and empirical issues', *Clinical Psychology Review*, 5, pp. 641-661.
Sheppard, B.H., Hartwick, J. and Warshaw, P.R. (1988), 'The theory of reasoned action: a meta-analysis of past research with recommendations for modifications and future research', *Journal of Consumer Research*, 15, pp. 325-343.
Sosa, R., Kennell, J., Klaus, M., Robertson, S. and Urrutia, J. (1980), 'The effect of a supportive companion on perinatal problems, length of labor and mother-infant interaction', *The New England Journal of Medicine*, 303, pp. 597-600.
Stern, J. (1983), 'Social mobility and the interpretation of social class mortality differentials', *Journal of Social Policy*, 12, pp. 27-49.
Tesser, A. and Shaffer, D.R. (1990), 'Attitudes and attitude change', *Annual Review of Psychology*, 41, pp. 479-523.
Thoits, P.A. (1982), 'Conceptual, methodological, and theoretical problems in studying social support as a buffer against life stress', *Journal of Health and Social Behavior*, 23, pp. 145-59.
Vaile, M.S.B., Calnan, M., Rutter, D.R. and Wall, B. (1993), 'Breast cancer screening services in three areas: uptake and satisfaction', *Journal of Public Health Medicine*, 15, pp. 37-45.
Weinstein, N.D. (1980), 'Unrealistic optimism about future life events', *Journal of Personality and Social Psychology*, 39, pp. 806-820.

Weinstein, N.D. (1982), 'Unrealistic optimism about susceptibility to health problems', *Journal of Behavioral Medicine*, 5, pp. 441-460.

Whitehead, M. (1987), *The Health Divide: Inequalities in Health in the 1980s*, Health Education Council, London.

Wilkinson, R.G. (ed.) (1986), *Class and Health: Research and Longitudinal Data*. Tavistock, London.

Wilkinson, R.G. (1994), 'Divided we fall: the poor pay the price of increased social inequality with their health', *British Medical Journal*, 308, pp. 1113-1114.